RAW CHI

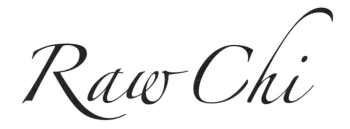

Raw Chi

Balancing the Raw Food Diet
with Chinese Herbs

———

Rehmannia Dean Thomas
Foreword by Janabai Owens-Amsden

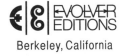

Berkeley, California

Published by Evolver Editions, an imprint of North Atlantic Books P.O. Box 12327 Berkeley, California 94712

Cover art © Marilyn Barbone/Shutterstock.com
Cover design by Brad Greene and Michael Robinson
Interior design by Brad Greene

All illustrations by Pablo Milberg and Rehmannia Dean Thomas except wrist pulse points illustration by Rehmannia Dean Thomas and splenic artery illustration in public domain. All photos by Rehmannia Dean Thomas.

Printed in the United States of America

MEDICAL DISCLAIMER: The following information is intended for general information purposes only. Individuals should always see their health care provider before administering any suggestions made in this book. Any application of the material set forth in the following pages is at the reader's discretion and is his or her sole responsibility.

Raw Chi: Balancing the Raw Food Diet with Chinese Herbs is sponsored by the Society for the Study of Native Arts and Sciences, a nonprofit educational corporation whose goals are to develop an educational and cross-cultural perspective linking various scientific, social, and artistic fields; to nurture a holistic view of arts, sciences, humanities, and healing; and to publish and distribute literature on the relationship of mind, body, and nature.

North Atlantic Books' publications are available through most bookstores. For further information, visit our website at www.northatlanticbooks.com or call 800-733-3000.

Library of Congress Cataloging-in-Publication Data

Thomas, Rehmannia Dean, 1957-
  Raw chi : balancing the raw food diet with Chinese herbs / by Rehmannia Dean Thomas ; foreword by Janabai Amsden.
    pages cm
  Summary: "Discusses chi in both men and women and presents Chinese herbs and tea recipes to supplement and balance diets high in raw foods"—Provided by publisher.
  ISBN 978-1-58394-858-3
  1. Raw food diet—Recipes. 2. Qi gong—Health aspects. 3. Herbs—Therapeutic use.
4. Tea—Therapeutic use. I. Title.
  RM237.5.T48 2014
  613.2'65—dc23
                                                                          2013044429

1 2 3 4 5 6 7 8 9 SHERIDAN 19 18 17 16 15 14
Printed on recycled paper

To my mother Joyce Adele Thomas and
my father Harold Edmond Thomas,
who help me write from the other side

_____

The breath of life moves through a deathless valley
Of mysterious motherhood
Which conceives and bears the universal seed,
The seeming of a world never to end,
Breath for men to draw from as they will;
And the more they take of it the more remains.

Lao Tzu, *The Way of Life According to Lao Tzu*, 6
—Translation by Witter Bynner

Great Taoist masters of ancient times developed the concepts I will discuss in this book. I consider myself merely a good interpreter of their philosophy. I am grateful that I was somehow chosen to spread this great wisdom to Western minds and that I am coming along with this information at what appears to be a perfect time to grasp the concepts at their depths. Shen Nong, Li Shizhen, Lao Tzu, and countless other wisdom seekers over many ages sought to understand life and its root mechanisims. Slowly but surely, they refined their empirical observations into a profound health lineage called the *Gate of Life* into which I have been initiated.

I am blessed to have received an eight-year apprenticeship under the renowned master herbalist Ron Teeguarden. He and his wife Yanlin, as well as his staff of knowledgeable doctors of traditional Chinese medicine whom I worked with side by side for nearly a decade, will always remain dear to my heart.

My ex-wife, Sharon Leong, initiated me into Eastern thinking when we went to China in 1985, where coincidentally, we visited many herb farms in Northeastern China (I did not then know Chinese herbology would become my profession). I remember how the people there revered the herbs, almost religiously, and now I know why. I am grateful for their subtle guidance and inspiration.

My new love of fifteen years, Michelle Wong, has further enlightened me on Eastern thinking and taught me how to use Microsoft Word to write my thoughts.

Many thanks to my awesome editor Terry Wolverton, whom I met through divine happenstance. Without her guidance I may never have produced any finished writing.

My parents are gone from this plane, but I do hope they can see this book. I'd like them to know something good came of the renegade kid they couldn't keep in Kentucky. And I have two cool brothers, Barry and Dave. I hope they know I love them.

CONTENTS

"Is tea raw?" That question did it. For a while, I had been an enthusiastic raw foodist as well as a follower of traditional Chinese medicine (TCM). But when a client of mine at Euphoria Loves Rawvolution asked about the large mason jar of herbal tea I was drinking, my thinking on these subjects began to solidify into something like a philosophy. I explained that tea is not raw. My client was genuinely surprised that I would drink a product that wasn't raw. I, in turn, was shocked that anyone's concept of healthy living would discard the ancient and worldwide healing tradition of herbal tea.

Raw food is the gift of Gaia, our Mother Earth, to humankind and all animals, great and small, through all time. The incredible healing power that raw food has on the human body is clear. Going raw cured me of a digestive disorder, made me lean and strong, granted me better sleep, provided me with new mental clarity, and afforded me an easy sense of peace. But not all raw foodists adhere to an all-or-nothing diet. For at least two thousand years, Chinese doctors have tested and perfected the art and science of TCM. In metaphoric terms, raw food is the hammer in healing, while Chinese medicine is the scalpel. In addition to the obvious benefits of loading your body with enzymes and nutrients in their original state, under the wise direction of TCM, you can also achieve a true and sustainable balance of health.

This seemed like a good theory to me, but I didn't have the knowledge of or experience with Chinese medicine to test my ideas. The practitioners I had met until then stuck to the "raw food is too cold for the body" line of thought.

Then one day, by complete surprise, the answer to my question materialized before me. I was visiting the Krishna Temple on Rose Avenue in Venice. When I arrived, my host stood on the sidewalk in deep discussion with another man. I introduced myself and learned that this man was Rehmannia, a Chinese herbalist who ran a weekly elixir bar at the Temple Lounge. Part cowboy and part medicine man, Rehmannia had a blend of casual yet practiced herbal wisdom.

Upon discussing the merits of raw food combined with Chinese medicine, we became instant kindred spirits. Excited to realize that we both agreed there could be a natural confluence between raw food and TCM, Rehmannia explained to me the concept of the "middle jiao" and the "triple warmer." He had designed an herbal formula for raw foodists to consume with meals. This formula would break the cycle of dampness and light the internal fires needed to boost kidney chi. My herbal prophet had arrived!

I was thrilled by his theory and invited him to put his formula into immediate action at our café. Within days we had Rehmannia's "Warming the Middle Jiao Tea" on tap at Euphoria Loves Rawvolution. Customers loved it, and we all started drinking it religiously with great results. All along, Rehmannia was there, checking our pulses to confirm his findings, delivering health lectures, serving teas, and imparting wisdom. Rehmannia is a true visionary in his ability to see through the collective dogma of the past and to the deeper teachings of TCM in order to serve the needs of the present.

I love raw foods. I know they are good for me. As debates go on endlessly about enzymes, phyto-nutrients, microbes, and digestion, those of us with lives to get on with just need to focus on eating the best food we can. I thrive on raw food and choose it whenever possible. I know it doesn't work for me in every season of the year and in every season of my life. I know from my cursory knowledge of Chinese medicine and Ayurvedic traditions that we are not the first generation to have wondered how to live and eat in balance with the world around us. And although our food and lifestyle options have grown exponentially, the search for true health is as old as disease itself.

TCM draws much of its ethos from the ancient philosophical and religious traditions of Taoism, which directs its practitioners to follow "the Tao" or "the Way" and to live in "naturalness," in balance with yin and yang, the polarities of the universal forces of masculine and feminine, darkness and light, the seen and the unseen. In the second century BC, a segment of Taoist tradition declared that the human body was a "microcosmos" that reflected the heavenly and ethereal planes. Like the firmament above, this microcosmos was governed by 36,000 gods and goddesses. These divine beings were in permanent residence within the body, guiding all inner hygienic processes. Believers were careful to eat healthfully, avoiding grains, meat, and wine to respect the inner gods and maintain a harmonious relationship with them.

Ancient Chinese doctors presaged science's recent discovery that our bodies are ruled by countless bacteria and that keeping their terrains healthy and functioning is the key to health for the individual. Caring for the whole organism requires cultivation and farming of the inner terrain through nurturing and supporting the numerous processes, patterns, and cycles within. TCM seeks to balance the health of the individual organism as a whole through a completely unique and infinitely customizable system that views the body as an ecosystem filled with elements, fluids, forces, and energy. Disease is perceived as a pattern of disharmony that is treated with a pantheon of herbs in specific combinations and sequences according to myriad variables based on the particular circumstances, patterns, and cycles for each individual patient.

Rehmannia's wonderful treatise on raw chi, in addition to making a powerful case for the inclusion of TCM into a raw diet, serves perhaps the unintended but defacto consequence of bringing the potential for inclusion of raw foods into Chinese medicine as well. Raw foods, previously disregarded by practitioners as too cold and damp, are now real possibilities for those who wish to follow the advice of Chinese herbalists while also exploring the healing power of raw food.

This book has brought to life not only the practice of TCM as an incisive diagnostic tool with an unlimited potential to heal, but it has also animated the human body as a breathing microcosmos, full of darkness and light, ebb and flow, mystery and illumination.

When I finished reading *Raw Chi* late at night, I was aware of my body as a living organism for the first time. I could feel the warmths, fluids, and energies of my personal *terroir* circulating and respirating. I was possessed by a powerful desire to breathe deeply and fill the alveoli of my lungs with the essential fuel my chi needs. I also knew without question that after my herbal tea the next morning, I would grab my raw kale, cucumbers, celery, and ginger to make a fresh juice, adding the vital nutrition that my body craved.

My life and my understanding of my own nature have changed profoundly after reading this book. The sacred wisdom and formulas it contains can instruct us all on how to more faithfully serve the 36,000 gods within.

JANABAI OWENS-AMSDEN
YEAR OF THE GREEN HORSE 4711

INTRODUCTION
The Flame of Life

"Life in all its fullness is Mother Nature obeyed."
—W. A. Price, from *Nutrition and Physical Degeneration*

Call it a fiery explosion, God's act or Mother's birth, fantasy dream or accidental happenstance. Whether from a bang or a gentle waking, whether elements swapping electrons or Brahma's out-breaths, our ideological boundaries converge in the belief that a pervasive energy spawned life and drives its evolution. The idea that this life had a birth and may someday end is what drives the curiosity of both religious mendicants and science-seekers.

Yet the origin of life is no better understood today than it has ever been. Our great seers and sages have pierced deep into life's ethericities (a term used by Viktor Schauberger to describe the ethereal energetic essences that he felt existed in the atmosphere). Great minds in science have brilliantly deciphered many of the physiological and unseen energetic mechanisms that drive life. Regardless, whence all this life was originally spawned and where it goes remains a mystery, albeit one that many of us feel is following a trajectory. We have terms for this—destiny, evolution, progress, refinement—and of course, we find ourselves tangled up within whichever web is being woven.

Long ago, ancient Chinese peoples cultivated a deep understanding of the principles that perpetuate life, and they accepted that life contained mysteries they could not explain. Over time they gleaned that creation is fueled by a not-yet-knowable master force that they called *chi*. This little, three-letter word packs a big punch. It encompasses many mechanical aspects of life's functions that have a close correlation with modern Western scientific theories. However, chi also accepts the as-yet unexplainable. As I will discuss in the coming pages, at the very root of chi is the *phrana*, the original breath of God.

Current Western science has lost sight of the *archana*, the magic or spirit behind life's alchemy, exactly the energetic aspect one of the Western fathers of medical chemistry, Paracelsus, warned against discarding. Today, for the most part, science views evolution as a purely materialistic and mechanical arrow shot from birth to death. Just about everything in our culture is designed to fit the idea that things begin at an A and calculably end at a Z. Science provides many enticing details about the nature of life—the periodic table of elements, for instance—but science mainly seeks to understand creation *once it has begun*. We know how electrons swap between the elements to create the mirage called life, but *what or who* does the swapping? The Chinese call it chi.

Explaining chi without getting bogged down in details is somewhat challenging. Fortunately for us Westerners, the Taoist masters, herbalists, and alchemists pierced to the core of life and used simple language to explain what they found. Therefore, we can go straight to the foundational ideology of Taoist health philosophy. Understanding these principles as traditional Chinese thinkers saw them can offer valuable insights about how to view life and maintain health.

Chi, the flame of life, gives rise to epochs and ecosystems and allows for their turning under to make way for new life. *All* life is beholden to this dynamic. Luckily, humans appear to have the option of learning something as we ride along. Maybe we'll be a little wiser when the end comes, if there is a finale, or maybe, like the Chinese thinkers have written, nothing is ever really finished and life keeps spiraling into infinity, rising out of itself and returning to rise again in a different shape.

The Chinese came to understand the essence of these cyclical patterns, not only in nature but in human physiology as well, and they formed a system to explain the flow of chi as a crucial requirement for the maintenance of health and vibrancy throughout all stages of our lives. Life's driving dynamic is located between two polarities the Chinese masters call *yin* and *yang*. When a dynamic equilibrium between these polarities is maintained, life is supported. If perfect balance is achieved, one will thrive, and quantum evolution will be possible. There are things we can do to help keep that balance. Do we want to grasp the reigns of our lives and grow older in harmonious health and vibrancy or languish in disempowerment and creep toward decrepitude?

Simply put, chi is the energy of change, and how it is *used* is the ultimate determiner of how life progresses. In the human body, life thrives when chi is flowing freely. Conversely, if chi is blocked or constricted, sickness and disease set in. This ideology is at the foundation of current Chinese medicine. It represents a principle that also applies to ciliates and pachyderm—everything that practices respiration and consumes carbon matter. But for the sake of economy, this book will focus on the flow of chi within humans, although I would like you to be mindful of how these principles apply to all life. Understanding this can change how you view existence and your part in it. Better health begets a better comprehension of life's experiences, and when chi is flowing with us instead of against us, we can more easily understand, embrace, and enhance our destinies, possibly even realize our highest potential. Through these we gain wisdom, and it all goes back around!

CHAPTER 1
Raw Energy

Approximately 5,000 years ago, wizened alchemists and herbalist-hermits lived in the high mountains of northern China. They breathed the forest air and looked to the sun. They listened to plant wisdom and ingested plant and animal parts we now call herbs, and this sustained them. They recognized that these herbs helped organisms develop and thrive and gave them strength and perception. They came to call this life-giving essence chi, a force that is absorbed, inhaled, and ingested into our bodies. They saw that this energy is recirculated through life's rise, decay, and rise again, and that we (and all living organisms) must consistently receive and transform this energy in order to maintain health.

Chi can be likened to a checking account on which we must rely for incremental deposits and withdrawals. Thus, we must take in chi in momentary and daily installments through *gathering chi* as oxygen breathed into our lungs and *nutritive chi*, the ingestion of the life force invested in food and water. We must then transform those life forces into bodily and vibrational energy. The closest Western equivalent to this process is the Krebs cycle (sometimes called the citric acid cycle), which describes the transformation of food into energy through a complex chemical process that results in adenosine triphosphate, or ATP, our cellular energy source. There has been a great deal of recent scientific study of ATP and how it is produced, but the Chinese have known about this principle for many centuries. They called it chi.[1]

The diamagnetic energy of the earth is chi. Enzymes are chi.[2] Chi represents a higher threshold of energy manifestation. Chi is power; it is combustion and heat and the *process* of transformation. Author Oliver

Morton states, "Life is a flame with a memory."[3] He is referring to how the flame of chi transforms one substrate into another.

Chi represents our daily energy needs, but we must take a moment to discuss deeper ramifications in the chi equation.

The Deeper Energy: Jing

Fortifying chi will give us long, healthy lives. Moreover, it may increase our potential to exhibit the vitality necessary for contributing to human development and culture. When our chi is sufficiently supplemented through diet, breath, and lifestyle, our inner wellspring of vitality bubbles over. Bodily processes such as metabolism, endocrine function and balance, immune regulation, and adaptability are supplemented. This abundance equips us with the energy we need in our daily lives.

Chi life force constantly feeds an ancient and primal energy the Chinese masters call *original chi*. This essence is accumulated in the kidney meridian, a system comprising the kidneys and adrenals, and held as *jing*. The closest Western word to jing is "essence." Jing is basically saved chi held for future use, particularly in reproduction, creativity, and bodily and genetic integrity. The very center of this accumulation/distribution point corresponds with the solar plexus and is called the *Gate of Life*. This is the beginning point of *the microcosmic orbit*, the circulation of our destiny's potential, which travels up the spine from our reproductive organs to the crown *chakra* and back. This original chi must be cultivated, protected, and nurtured. It forms our base vitality and gives light to our aura. Genius can be born of the combination of jing and chi.

With strong chi and jing, our health is robust, and we enjoy satisfying adventures in the creative and procreative realms. We may experience youthful vitality well into our older years. Jing is our family genetic gold vault, which contains the epigenetic energy of our ancestors and which our great grandchildren will inherit. Everything we do, think, and eat during our lives will be imbedded in the jing of our progeny. How much of this gold are you spending, and how much are you saving?

If we receive insufficient chi from poor diet, breathing, and lifestyle, we may drag ourselves around at half speed, using stimulants like coffee and sugar to turn up our chi fire and get a temporary boost. These stimulants and simple, fast-burning sugars provide a temporary energy the Chinese call "false fire" and trigger the body's endocrine system to produce energy that is not the true energy derived from chi's ethericities. If this deficiency is not corrected, we will begin to draw on the deeper reserves of our jing to get through the day. Using jing in lieu of true chi energy will begin draining our gold vault—rendering us vulnerable at our genetic base. When this precious essence of jing is "leaked," we will lose our sense of adventure and age more rapidly. If we continue to live this way, we will pass on "pre-natal jing deficiency" to our children, which can lessen their vitality. Thus, the Chinese have a saying: "It is okay to feel fatigued (chi depleted) but not exhausted (jing and chi depletion)," for chi is an incremental energy that we must take in on a regular basis.

We need to support chi at all times through a diet high in life-giving foods and herbs along with good breathing, sunlight, and a healthy lifestyle, so our jing will remain fortified.

If our energy is drained, we can make a quick deposit by taking deep breaths of air, eating nutritious food prepared so that it retains its inherent chi, and taking herbs imbued with deep chi and jing empowerment. When fresh, incoming chi maintains a full jing gold vault, we will live in optimal and versatile self-empowerment.

Jing is our code of replication and restoration, like a stone tablet of information. Chi is the process of applying that information. Jing is the reproductive potential; chi is the force that activates the production of new life from the old. Chi must be derived from good fuel. We should warm the house with oak logs in the fireplace, not wads of newspaper. Chi is the cutting and stacking of the logs and the stoking of a good fire to warm the hearth, while jing represents the extra logs you mindfully stored for the winter. Jing is even the stones and mortar of the fireplace itself.

Maintaining chi and jing will help assure the adrenals can quickly recuperate from the stresses of life and remain vital. Through healthy adrenals, we maintain impetus and energy, including a healthy stress response, integrity of the musculature framework, quick mental response, balanced immune response, creativity, adventure, and the good old libido. Furthermore, when the blood is coursing with these vital essences, the heart will be nourished and the brain will receive *upright chi*, which nourishes the perception of our higher selves and our true potential. The following illustration depicts the original gathering of chi and its conversion into energy, both for immediate use and for a supply to be stored in the kidneys for future use.

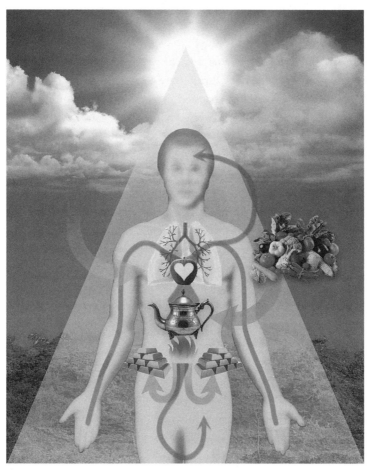

Our personal gold vault of health is kept full by the gathering of true chi.

CHAPTER 2
Gathering Chi

The dynamics of light set into action the energy we call the *original chi,* which fuels photosynthesis, vitamin synthesis, and all forms of metamorphic and catabolic action. The ancient mystics of India and China said that another original source of chi is held in the *phrana,* or breath, and is gathered in the lung alveoli when oxygen molecules enter red blood cells, giving mobility to the blood. This helps warm the body and circulate vital energy. It might also explain why we see so many young women in yoga class at 7 a.m.; they are gathering chi as oxygen into the bloodstream so that they have energy for the coming day.

Nutritive chi is derived from our diet. Foods are bundles of energy. These substrate materials are carbon based, and as carbon is the most highly dynamic element in nature, it can manifest as the whole cornucopia and pharmacopoeia in our kitchens and medicine cabinets. Carbohydrates—sugars, fats, and starches—and all proteins, animal and vegetable, are carbon material, and mineral ions are meshed among them. How we assimilate these materials determines the degree of our daily and long-term vitality.

Foods in their natural state contain protein-based packets of chi waiting to be unleashed. These are called enzymes. Enzymes are nature's catalysts; they speed up the conversion of biogenic processes and are found in all living material. Enzyme-rich foods contain their own agents to transform rough materials into chi; this makes it easier for the human body to digest these foods. Conversely, the enzymes in food are wiped out by heavy cooking and processing. The digestive organs must produce extra enzymes and hormones to digest them, making them work harder to extract nutrients for the body's daily energy needs.

This is the primary argument in favor of eating foods raw or foods carefully cooked with low heat. Enzymes begin to be destroyed at temperatures as low as 108 degrees, and food is generally cooked at much higher temperatures.

Some people have figured this out, and a burgeoning movement is taking place among raw food enthusiasts. These people understand the simple and obvious fact that we have been destroying the value of our food through cooking and processing, thus depriving ourselves of true nutrition through processes that prioritize making food look appetizing and taste good over protecting its chi. (In subsequent chapters, I will discuss how the cooking of certain foods, including some starches and proteins, helps prepare these nutrients for easier extraction by the body.) The crown of an energetic food pyramid is occupied by fresh foods that are grown well in highly nutrient-fortified soils, eaten raw or carefully prepared, and chosen according to season.

So does this mean that the raw food diet is the answer to all our problems? Partially, yes, provided we do our homework to ensure we derive the full spectrum of nutrients that we need for our individual health. However, there are a few potential dangers that may accompany a diet high in raw foods as well. Many vegetables and fruits are considered yin foods, and are thus potentially dampening to the organs and glands that regulate chi. This can definitely present problems, particularly for women, and most particularly for those who live in colder climates or who suffer from excess moisture retention, cold hands and feet, and anemia and/or excessive menstrual bleeding. I have written this book to explore a remedy for these potential drawbacks.

Yin Foods: Cooling and Dampening

Many of us interested in the raw food diet have had the experience of visiting our acupuncturist and seeing a finger waving in our faces. "No raw food. Damp spleen!" What exactly is the acupuncurist talking about? The prevailing thought in Chinese medicine is that raw foods are too cooling and dampening for some people, especially women, to properly digest and from which to derive sufficient chi.

I first heard about the raw food movement in 2003 and quickly took my questions to a doctor of Chinese medicine I had worked with under my teacher Ron Teeguarden.

Me: What do think about the raw food diet?

Him: Not a good idea.

Me: Why not?

Him: Too cold. Vegetables and fruits are cooling and watery. They will cause edema around the middle *jiao* (abdomen) and dampen the spleen, which is governor of chi.

Okay, I could believe that. I'd been studying how the Chinese view digestion as governed by a system that they merely call the "spleen" but that actually includes the stomach, pancreas, duodenum, and small intestine. The Chinese believe the spleen system (which we will look at in detail in chapter three) must remain dry and warm in order to fortify red and white blood cells and govern the metabolism of food. I knew this health wisdom had been gained through empirical observation over centuries.

Yet somehow my gut told me there was something good in the raw food diet (albeit not exclusively). I felt there must be a harmonious equation to engage these two views. I wanted to get some answers.

My first insight walked in the door not long after. A young woman sauntered up to the elixir bar I was managing under Master Teeguarden (inventor of the modern elixir bar) in Santa Monica, California. She sat at a barstool, erect and proud. I'd say she was in her mid-twenties. Her eyes were bright and her mind very quick, except that she displayed a jittery and talkative nature; she was ungrounded and had difficulty focusing. The Chinese believe many young Americans exhibit this "windy" energy. Her skin was well-pigmented and radiantly healthy, but she had pretty bad acne, some of the pimples very large. Her body was toned and agile, yet she had distention around her abdomen and hips.

As we talked, she proudly declared she was a strict raw foodist. I had been curious about the pulse of someone on a raw food diet, and here

11

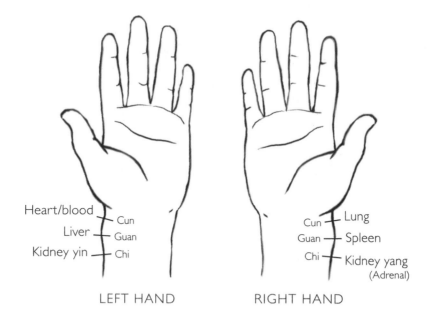

Heart/blood — Cun	Cun — Lung
Liver — Guan	Guan — Spleen
Kidney yin — Chi	Chi — Kidney yang (Adrenal)

LEFT HAND   RIGHT HAND

was my first subject. My fellow herbalists had said those on a raw food diet may show a weak pulse at the spleen point (located at the center or *guan* point on the right wrist, where the terminal point of the radius bone protrudes just below the ball of the thumb metacarpal bone)...

I asked to take her pulse, and it was *very* strong! In fact, stronger than the majority of women I'd checked before, even those on conscientious omnivorous diets. I asked to view her tongue. It was healthy but somewhat pale and bloated with slight teeth marks along the edges—indicators that are associated with damp spleen. Yet her pulse was thriving! This meant her spleen/pancreas was working quite well as governors of the digestion and metabolism of her food, but there were also signs of inner dampness.

I went home and thought about this. How could she have abundant energy, a curious and extroverted personality, and a strong spleen pulse, while at the same time displaying signs of *chi stagnation*—her pale tongue, acne, and slightly widening hips? I suspected there was a way to augment her raw food diet in order to avoid these symptoms, and I soon found it. Strangely, it had been right under our noses all along—in the herbal formulas sitting on the shelf at Dragonherbs.

Various classic herbal formulas derived from the Chinese *Materia medica* have been developed over centuries to help dry the spleen/pancreas and assist chi in metabolizing and assimilating energy into the body. Chi-enhancing formulas, which have been renowned for their effectiveness in warming the middle jiao, have been well-tested over time, but these formulas have been generally utilized to treat *already* accumulated dampness and edema associated with weak spleen/digestion. Had anyone considered these herbal formulas as adjuncts in the daily diet to help *prevent* moisture retention and bodily cooling? I guessed not.

Master Teeguarden had us study the Chinese Pharmacopoeia of herbs, which contained a category on chi herbs. These herbs are said to warm the digestion and assist metabolism of food into energy and blood. I found that many of these herbs are considered harmless for daily use when taken properly in conjunction with other herbs. The herbal formulas had been meticulously crafted over centuries to assist spleen chi, and these too appeared to be safe for daily consumption. Could this girl, and others who eat raw food, take these herbal formulas on a daily basis to support chi? After some ruminating, I felt assured that these kinds of herbal formulas could work well as a daily adjunct to the raw food diet; they could truly assist chi and help *prevent* accumulation of unwanted moisture retention. Hot tea taken along with raw foods . . .

I mulled and researched some more and eventually went to my herbalist cohort to ask what he thought.

Me: I'm thinkin' that spleen chi tonics could be taken along with the raw food diet as an adjunct to *prevent* cooling and water retention, rather than merely using the herbal formulas *after* damp spleen and bloating has occurred.

Him: Hmmm . . . you could be right.

I asked some other Chinese doctors and got a contemplative nod of approval from each of them. Thus began the thinking that led to this book.

CHAPTER 3
Yin and Yang of Chi

In Eastern ideology, evolution is thought to progress in a series of spirals, each one rising slightly higher than the one before it, resembling a spring from which new life can emerge.

Ancient Chinese men and women looked upon nature from their hillside caves and saw cycles of hot/dry and cold/wet. They saw night and day, that the sun progressed through longer and shorter days, creating seasons that led back to each other. They came to recognize a dynamic balancing act of two opposing forces that governed life as we know it, two polarities held in a dynamic equilibrium. Life appeared to sit delicately upon the crux of an energetic seesaw between these two extremes. These wise men and women concluded that all forces of life must be held within the balance of this dynamic equipoise. If one extreme over powered or disabled the other, and/or the opposing energies split apart, all life would end.

These ancient people drew a diagram in which two teardrops swim around each other within a circle. The teardrops are equal in size and shape. One represents exertion, thrust, heat, and day, the other, rest, night, coolness, wetness. One teardrop represented the time when the heat came, the fruits and tubers grew sweet, and the canopy of green cast cooling shade over the people's huts. The days were long, and the people arose earlier and hunted longer. During the time symbolized by the other teardrop, the days were shorter, and the people rested longer in their caves. They stayed out of the bitter cold and hunted less. The white snows came, and the once tufty trees in the forest dropped their leaves and stood naked, their skeletal arms reaching up in search of the sun. The white winds blew, and everything seemed to retreat to shiver in nooks and crannies. The people wondered if it all had died. How could anything live out there?

But the warm breezes came again, and the trees sprouted their green tufts. Everything returned as it had been before, when the animals, fruits, and herbs were plentiful. Everything hadn't died after all! Life, death, and new life followed each other in cycles. The drawing of the two teardrops explained these cycles for the people of the mountain. They made a very important observation, one that forms the cornerstone for understanding the dynamic of chi and of all life. But this drawing didn't represent the complete picture; something was missing.

The ancient people continued to observe nature's cycles of growth, decay, and regrowth. They came to understand that energy didn't only manifest as opposing forces in a constant tug of war; this was too extreme. There had to be a little of the opposite energy within each teardrop for the whole to maintain balance. When the cold, white winds came, and the leaves withered and fell, the forest didn't die in the process. Perhaps a small pilot light of life still burned within, so that the next season could begin. The dormant period of rest and stasis—which these people called yin—contained within it the seed of yang, waiting to initiate the next growing season. These insightful people saw that when the hot days came and the forest was full, they needed a few cool rains and cool nights, or everything would become too dry and fires would burn in the forest. The yang period of warmth and acceleration needed to have that little yin balance, or it would consume itself.

The ancients then examined their own patterns and survival needs and found that on hot days, they needed to take more water on their hunting and gathering treks; they needed to stop and rest a while in the shade. On the cold, white days, they needed to kindle the fire hearth for warmth. When they slept at night, they didn't die; a little pitter patter was still going on in their chests.

Thus, these early people of the mountains of northern China drew two little dots of the opposite color within the two larger teardrops, describing life. Yin and yang were held in perfect equipoise via these two little dots; these nuclei generated the cyclical flow of yin and yang. In this way, the fires wouldn't come, and the white winds would eventually recede. Life would thrive and transform itself into new life.

The symbol of yin and yang became the foundation of Chinese health philosophy. The ancients had realized a truth, that by keeping these forces in balance, chi would remain vibrant. Conversely, when the balance of yin and yang is upset, chi may stagnate or consume itself. These are the mechanisms of illness and disease. During yin time, what if the white winds remained too long? The pilot light might be extinguished, and new life might not be triggered. In the yang time, what if the rains and cool nights didn't come? Fires might start and consume everything. Thus, yin and yang must balance each other for life to thrive. The same is true in the microcosm of our bodies. The flame of metabolism must be fanned, and the wellspring of our future must be filled. When these are held in balance, we enjoy the gift of health.

The Five Organ Meridians

By approximately 1500 BC, the Chinese had developed a surprisingly accurate understanding of human physiology and metabolism, including reproductive and neurological endocrinology. They perceived the body as containing five primary organ systems that must work in harmonious interaction for health to be maintained. These *functional* networks contain yin and yang organ meridians and other components—the heart, liver, lung, kidney, and spleen meridians. We will briefly look at these organ systems and their primary times of dominance so that we can better understand the functions of the two primary organ/gland systems that "govern" chi within the *milieu intérieur** of the human body: the lung (gathering chi) system and the spleen (nutritive chi) system.

The ancient Chinese health mendicants drew a diagram of the four organ systems that they referred to as interdependent functional "meridians" on the north, south, east, and west perimeters, with the spleen

*A term coined by French Physician Claude Bernard (1813–1878) while studying the beneficial role of probiotic bacteria in the human digestive system.

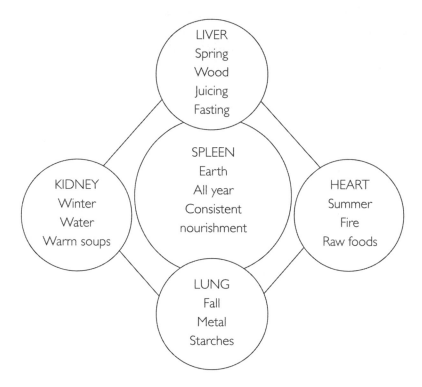

meridian occupying a position in the middle. This was their way of associating the spleen meridian with the element *earth*, which is in the center of our cosmology. The four seasons are associated with four of the five organ systems, but the spleen system is not linked to any particular season. This is because it is seen as requiring "tonification," consistent support, throughout the year.

The spleen meridian includes the stomach, spleen, pancreas, duodenum, and small intestine. These organs and glands comprise a functional unit that governs our metabolism.

The other four organ systems are dominant during certain times of the day and the year. For instance, spring begins with the liver meridian, which includes the gallbladder. In spring we need to cleanse the blood and liver by fasting on clean water and the juices of fresh, raw vegetables and grasses. We can lose a little weight during this time and take cleansing, herbal tonics to help remove unwanted yeasts and other microbes from the bloodstream. In Chinese ideology, the liver is associated with the element *wood.* The liver is dominant during the late night hours, 1–3 a.m.

In summer we must take care of our heart, as the hot weather is upon us, and we can get heated inside. This is the period when the cooling vegetables of summer ripen, and our diet may be comfortably raw. The heart meridian includes the pericardium and the arterial and vascular network and is associated with the element *fire.* The heart meridian is dominant during the hottest time of day: 11 a.m.–1 p.m.

During fall the Chinese say we must protect our lungs from the cooler, drier fall winds that kick up carcinogenic dusts. This is the time to carry a scarf and tie it around your nose and mouth while riding your bike! Our root vegetables ripen; our starchy foods—potatoes, squash, and onions—are ready for consumption. We can take herbal teas that include magnolia bud, licorice root, and cordyceps. These foods help warm our bodies and can aid in adding a little extra cellulose padding as we prepare for winter. The lung meridian is comprised of the lung and large intestine.

Starchy vegetables should be carefully cooked, as the starches are not easily digestible in their raw state; they are best "gelatinized" or lightly roasted for easier assimilation into the body. At this time we should modify our raw diet and allow a few cooked starches into our meals. The lung meridian is associated with the element *metal* and is dominant from 3 a.m.–5 a.m.

Winter is dominated by the kidney meridian, which includes the adrenals. We sleep longer, stay inside by the fire, and nurture ourselves so that we can restore our adrenals. We want to drink hot, soothing drinks and take our proteins in the form of soups and stocks. Lentil soup, barley and minestrone soup, oatmeal, dhal, miso soup, black bean soup, etc., are beneficial during this time, as are lightly steamed winter vegetables like pumpkin and squash. You can let yourself gain a few pounds, because you're going to fast or cleanse when the spring comes. Drink hot tea during this time and take elixirs that include kidney-tonifying herbs such as ho shou wu, schizandra, goji, and rehmannia glutinosa (prepared). Kidney essence is associated with the element *water*. The kidneys are dominant during the hours 5–7 p.m.

As mentioned, the spleen meridian is the governor of chi. This is where old blood is stripped down and some of the body's new blood is built. While traveling through the other organs and glands of the spleen system, blood attains the vital freshness to hold and carry chi. Of course, all five organ systems work in tandem to maintain a healthy body, and there are confounding details in attempting to fully explain blood physiology. The liver, kidneys, and bone marrow are all involved in blood maintenance, so let us look briefly into the sojourn of chi through the body before further examining the physiology of the spleen meridian. There we will hopefully gain clarity on why the Chinese believe this organ meridian is specific to the production of chi.

CHAPTER 4
Chi Is Carried in the Blood

Vitalization of the blood begins with gathering chi, when the lungs infuse the body with oxygen. When this happens, oxygen molecules—a primary blood mobilizer—attach to blood cells. The oxygen helps the body break down carbohydrates into glucose (blood sugar) to be used as food for cellular metabolism. From there the blood begins its distribution away from the heart through the arterial network. From the aortal artery, blood is siphoned into the celiac trunk and to the splenic arterial system, where it travels through the walls of the stomach, pancreas, duodenum, and spleen. Through actions in the splenic system and in the liver and bone marrow, oxygen molecules in the blood cells bind with iron ions. A myriad of heme proteins surrounds the iron ions to protect the cell from the iron's potential toxicity. At that point, the blood cell has attained what is called hemoglobin—the carrier of vital chi to the cells, tissues, and organs.

The blood then passes through the splenic vein to the liver for more chemical reactions, fat storing, and blood cleansing and then carries the nutrients and oxygen to the cells, allowing the body to store energy in such forms as adenosine triphosphate (ATP).

The sustenance of chi is a two-way street; in order to infuse the blood with vital energy, the organs that govern the maintenance of chi must be nourished with foods of high nutritive value that are well assimilated. In return, this vitalized blood keeps the body warm and animated. The Chinese have a saying: "Blood is the mother of chi, and chi follows blood."

Exactly how the blood comes to hold chi forms the crux of our discussion. When there is no chi in the blood, there is also no metabolic and catabolic activity. Chi stagnation will set in, and unless cleared, disease may follow.

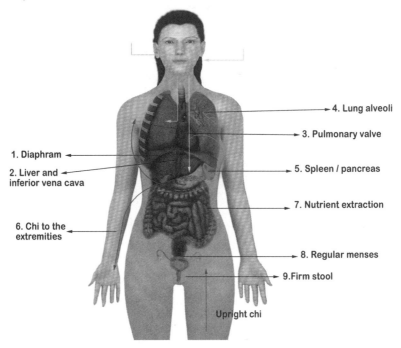

1. Diaphram
2. Liver and inferior vena cava
6. Chi to the extremities

4. Lung alveoli
3. Pulmonary valve
5. Spleen / pancreas
7. Nutrient extraction
8. Regular menses
9. Firm stool

Upright chi

In the above drawing we see that oxygen, referred to as gathering chi, is brought into the body. During an inhalation (1), the diaphragm pushes down on the liver and kidneys, helping to press old, deoxygenated blood (2) into the inferior vena cava, which acts as the main transport vessel of deoxygenated blood upward from the lower part of the body, while the superior vena cava returns blood to the heart from the head and arms. The blood is then pumped (3) through the pulmonary valve of the heart and diffused into capillaries surrounding the lung alveoli (4), where it is saturated with oxygen. This starts the process of blood vitalization. The blood then begins its sojourn toward the various organs via the arterial system.

According to Chinese medicine, the blood's next major stop on the chi highway occurs via the splenic artery, which splits off of the celiac trunk from the aortal artery just below the heart. The splenic arterial network brings blood to the walls of the stomach and courses through the pancreas, supporting this gland's important enzyme-producing activity. Also during this passage, the blood is filtered and vitalized in the spleen, where it receives nutritive chi from the duodenum and small intestine (5). This is where ingested foods are "cooked down" and infused with vital chi energy. The splenic vascular system carries the blood toward the liver for cleansing, filtering, and more fortification. (Nutritive chi may also be derived via the mesenteric arterial and vascular networks to and from the large intestine, but the Chinese do not believe this to be part of the spleen meridian.)

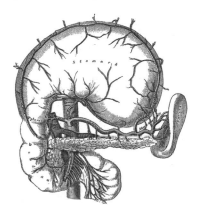

Arteries of the spleen meridian feeding blood to the walls of the stomach, pancreas, spleen, duodenum, and small intestine

The Chinese believe that after the blood has received its *mobilizer*, oxygen, and its *fortifier*, new ferrous iron, along with an array of heme proteins, it is fully infused with chi. Once this has been achieved, the blood can carry oxygen and nutrients to the cells and organs. The body has upright chi, with vital blood flowing freely to the head, arms, and legs (6) and back toward the heart through the vascular system. With sufficient chi, the food we've eaten will be fully cooked down, the middle jiao of the body will maintain a warm flame, and extra moisture will be "steamed off" by the digestive process. The walls of the intestines will be ready to extract more nutrients (7), and proper body weight will be maintained. Women will have regular and pain-free menstrual cycles (8), and all of us will have daily stools (9) of semifirm waste.

Chi is enhanced by the conscious eating of food. Slowing down and thoroughly chewing food is essential. Salivation of well-chewed food also provides enzymes that aid the process of chi extraction in the stomach. Gulping down insufficiently chewed food makes it hard for the body to extract chi. Likewise, overcooking food kills the enzymes nature has provided to aid our digestion. Whole, raw, plant-based foods contain enzymes that assist digestive breakdown and nutrient extraction.

CHAPTER 5

The Spleen: Valve of the Driving Force

The Chinese view the five organ meridians as units of interdependent function, comprising major and minor organs and glands. Their collective efficiency is regarded over the specific functions of each organ/gland in the system. The spleen system consists of the stomach, spleen, pancreas, duodenum, and small intestine, which act like a stovetop burner located under the pot of soup or tea that is the stomach.

Nutritive chi begins with the mixing of saliva into foods while in the mouth, where the first digestive enzymes are introduced, and continues with the passage of food through the esophagus. Reaching the stomach, the food "bolus" (masticated and salivated meal) is churned and infused with secretions including hydrochloric acid, pepsin, and mucus, which are secreted through the stomach wall, and break down the ingested food into a "hydrolyzed" soup, a semiliquid called chyme. During this process, enzymes from the pancreas secrete into the stomach to help break down any other substrate materials, such as proteins, starches, and minerals, and render their nutrients absorbable into the body.

Once this stage is finished, a sphincter at the bottom end of the stomach opens and allows the chyme of soupy material to enter the first part of the intestine, the duodenum. Here ducts from the gallbladder inject bile into the mesh, and a myriad of other chemical reactions take place to further cleave and break down any resilient fats, proteins, and starches. These and other chemicals realkalinize the pH of the chyme, reducing the hydrochloric acid so that the food doesn't enter the small intestine in a highly acidic state (which would cause some pretty bad indigestion). The duodenum also supplies fresh ferrous iron to be taken up in the red blood.

At this stage, the inherent pH of the ingested foods can affect our health. If the foods we eat create acidity in the body, as do many of the standard foods eaten in the United States (i.e., meat, dairy, sugar), many more stomach acids and pancreatic enzymes will be needed to digest the food. This requires the gallbladder and duodenum to secrete more chemicals to safely alkalinize this mix, lest again, we should experience major pain in our middle jiao. In this phase, the chyme is "spit" back and forth through the sphincter of the duodenum and stomach to thoroughly infuse the mixture with the necessary chemicals for digestion. This and earlier stomach peristalsis causes the gurgling we sometimes hear coming from our stomachs.

Vegetarian and raw food diets are mainly composed of foods whose pH is alkaline or alkaline *forming*, such as citrus fruits. Yet excessive (hyper-alkalinity) alkalinity in the blood and other body fluids is also dangerous. The body, in its amazing intelligence, manages to maintain a pH just above the midway point between acid and alkaline—just slightly alkaline—at approximately 7.4 on a scale of 14. Sickness can occur when the body's pH strays from this perimeter, the most common ailments of our society occurring when the pH drifts toward acidity.

Now broken down into this meshy soup, its pH alkalinized, the food seeps into the small intestine, where its nutrients are absorbed through the intestinal walls and into the blood cells. Up to 95 percent of nutrient absorption occurs through the walls of the small intestine when arteries associated with the splenic artery bring blood to the area. From there, the blood is drawn back through the splenic vascular system and then heads toward the liver.

The liver, bone marrow, and kidneys also play important roles in blood building, cleansing, and fortification, but for the sake of conciseness, we will focus on the splenic system in this book.

Why did the ancient Chinese believe the spleen meridian governs digestive metabolism? They saw that the spleen contains a reservoir of red and white blood cells. The white blood cells phagocytize (destroy) old, spent red blood cells in the spleen, and fresher blood leaves via the splenic vein. Therefore, the Chinese came to view the spleen as the site where octane is infused into the body's fuel. In this regard, they were right: only fresh, vital blood leaves the spleen and commences its journey through the other organs of the splenic system. This blood has more capacity to absorb and deliver nutrients and minerals and to carry oxygen to the body's cells and organs. The Chinese looked "upstream" to discover where blood's vitality is monitored. The spleen is the beginning point; while sifting through the spleen, the blood is "tailored" to draw in new chi.

The spleen's reservoir of defensive white blood cells infuse the blood with *protective chi;* they are our immune cells. These white blood cells need to be very aggressive in order to fend off the invasion of *pathogenic chi,* including yeast colonization, mutated or damaged cells, and viral infestation. These large white cells also scavenge microbes, protids, and other unwanted stuff in the plasma, lymph, and other humors (an old medical term for any and all bodily fluids).

Without the spleen, the body is not as well-equipped to revitalize blood and infuse it with defensive properties. Since red blood is mainly produced in bone marrow (with some produced in the liver), it is possible to live without a spleen, but under these circumstances, one runs a risk of infection, due to a lesser immune system. Such people should strive to maintain a diet that is more alkaline and high in living foods and enzymes. The raw food diet will benefit them, provided they keep warm in the middle jiao. These people should thoroughly chew foods and seek infusions of new blood into the body once in a while. They should also avoid immune-compromising foods that have allergenic properties.

The issue of blood vitality and maintenance, as well as the regulation of sufficient ratios of red blood in the body, is of central importance in the maintenance of chi. Blood deficiency is a potential problem for women, due to monthly blood loss during menstruation. I will discuss this further in chapter eight.

Failing to provide the blood with essential chi because of insufficient dietary habits will deprive the body of the essential nutrients needed for health.

Spleen Chi Deficiency

If we do not eat wholesome foods, the spleen chi becomes deficient, resulting in a sluggish metabolism. The quality of the fuel we consume is vitally
important. Today many industrialized farming practices rely on "forcing"
food to grow through excessive irrigation and the use of inorganic fertilizers that are high in nitrogen. Chemicals are mainly used to protect the
crops from weed invasion and damage from pests. This mass production
of chemical-laced food grown with inorganic fertilizers and heavy irrigation results in leached and depleted soils. The chemicals kill beneficial
microorganisms in the soil and eventually rob it of essential nutrients and
elements, including humic and fulvic acids, precisely the microorganisms
that make the soil's minerals available to plants. Though these foods wind
up on our grocery shelves looking nice and green, they may be deficient
in nutrients and minerals.

Further diminution occurs when food is harvested before it is ripe, a
necessity in our current long-distance food distribution system. In addition, the over-processing of our foods—which is done primarily to increase
shelf life and provide so-called "convenience" for the consumer—renders
much of our food nutritionally deficient. There isn't any chi in this food,
which causes our engines to slow down and run sluggishly.

Weak spleen chi is prevalent in our society because of the devital-
ized foods on our tables. If the fuel we're taking in is lacking in enzymes
and other metabolic catalysts, the spleen system will not be able to function at the pace necessary to transform food into energy (ATP). Without
the proper infusion of chi, the digestive temperature may cool. Water and
dampness may not be steamed off and may instead accumulate, causing the
spleen organs to become damp. This results in an inability to metabolize
fats, liquids, and estrogen; is associated with fluid retention at the cellular
level; and inhibits the extraction of nutrients from our food.

The accumulation of water around the hips, which occurs more often
with women than men, is a sign of damp spleen. This is very common in
the United States. Spleen chi deficiency causes a chain reaction in which
we put on extra pounds but remain hungry; our bodies suffer from mal-
nutrition even though we are gaining weight! This makes it difficult for

women to maintain proper blood and estrogen levels, metabolize water and fat, and maintain hormonal balance and a healthy thyroid. Many women, particularly in their thirties, endure the distressing malady of widening hips even while engaging in excessive exercise, all the while thinking it is fat they are inexplicably accumulating. In many cases, fluid retention, or edema, may be the actual culprit. We will discuss this in detail in the next chapter.

Men also accumulate dampness from weak spleen chi. This condition in men usually manifests as a warm, damp, phlegmatic buildup around the digestive region. In addition to the stomach bloating outward, this causes bacterial, fungal, parasitic, and other metabolic problems for men.

The inability of the body to extract chi, or anabolic fuel elements during digestion can cause people to start dipping into their deeper reserves of jing (mentioned in chapter two) in order to get through the day. Metaphorically, when you have drained the checking account (chi) and begun dipping into the savings account (jing), you are chipping away at your future security. We must nourish ourselves with chi-building whole foods and herbs to avoid using the vital jing essence for our daily energy needs. When people eat foods insufficient in life force, they may have to tap into their adrenal reserves to get by. The adrenals are like a portal into the jing reserves; therefore, using them for energy causes rapid aging. Overwork; stress; excessive sexual activity, sexual suppression, and menstrual bleeding; illnesses; and accidents can also lead to excessive adrenal activity. The energy from the adrenals is called "false fire" and should be avoided. Tapping this finite and insufficient source for long-term energy needs will cause a chronic lack of vitality at our root—a lack of creativity, adventure, libido, general metabolism, and mental alertness and lead to a host of deficiency diseases.

It all begins with how well we breathe and the quality of the food we eat.

CHAPTER 6
Raw Foods, Herbs, and Chi: Understanding the Equation

The raw food movement is vital and important, but there are some potential detriments to a raw food diet. Modification is the message nowadays. I hope this book will provide information that can assist not just raw food mendicants who wish to adhere to their strict principles of a raw-only diet but others as well. Regardless of how much cooked or raw food you eat, these principles can help you to maintain a diet that supports chi and, thus, health.

Raw, uncooked foods are classified as yin, which means they are watery and cooling to the system; they exert a dampening effect on the metabolic functions. Most women have what is called a "yin constitution." They can hold excess moisture and are prone to experiencing the undesirable aspects and after effects of extensive raw, yin food consumption.

There is a great deal of available information on foods, their phytochemistry, and actions, so I will refrain from lengthy discussions of those subjects here and instead relay a few observations regarding sourcing, food chemistry, and metabolism to clarify certain aspects of chi.

Sourcing Foods High in Chi

As mentioned before, mass food production depends on chemicals and processes, like pesticides and excessive irrigation, that deplete food of nutrients and, thus, chi. Organic farming can also rob foods of chi. Much organic farming is done on very large plots of land with machinery. The lack of biodiversity on these farms affects soil fertility, as it is difficult to disperse sufficient composted biomass on these large parcels of land. And the machines used to propagate and harvest these plants do not allow a human "imprint" to be imbued to the plants during cultivation.

Surely, the small farmers who work with hand tools and maintain on-site compost piles, who bless and fortify their soil for our benefit should be hailed as our society's saviors. My friend Jerry Price is one of those blessed farmers. I have met many small farmers who took great pride in knowing they were providing true sustenance for their community. True farmers are generally inherently spiritual, hearing the sound of Earth's voice, and they are often-times far more versed in the socio-political goings-on of the world and understand the residual impact our actions have down the food chain to their soil and our health. I try to shop for vegetables at small, local farmers markets. I look for people at the stalls who have dirt under their fingernails, and I ask how large their farm is. If it is two acres or fewer, I will buy the vegetables. On a farm this small, the farmhands will more likely be able to keep the soil composted, and the plants will be cared for by humans, rather than by chemicals.

But of course, the very best way to produce your food is in your backyard or a nearby community garden. I grow lots of unsightly weeds in my garden, sometimes perplexing my gardening neighbors, but I tell them there's more chi in those weeds! The more that humans culti-vate plants, the more they may potentially reduce the plants' inherent jing. Making it easy for a plant to thrive will allow the plant to stop producing many phytochemicals that it needs in order to survive in the wild, therefore depriving ourselves of these valuable nutrients and plant medicines.

Gut Flora Assist Chi and Blood

For economy, I will not engage in a detailed dissertation on gut flora, for there are many other sources for this information. But it is valuable to state that gut flora are intrinsically involved in the digestion and assimilation of the myriad structures of nutrients and minerals from our food. In particular, they are indispensable in rendering iron assimilable to red blood cells. In fact, they could be considered part of the spleen meridian. Consuming raw foods high in chi supports these alkaline-loving bacteria and helps supply the new, beneficial bacteria that have not been destroyed by cooking. These bacteria promote a healthy body pH by encouraging the fermentation of foods while passing through the digestive tract. Conversely, harmful bacteria can build up in our guts and allow the putrification of foods while in the intestines. This will swing the body's pH toward acidity. The destruction of friendly bacteria by antibiotics and the proliferation of harmful, acid-loving bacteria and other microbes from excessive consumption of acid-forming, over-cooked, and sugary foods (like those in the standard American diet), can disrupt proper digestion. This bacterial imbalance, "called dysbiosis," is now being indicated in many maladies, including leaky gut[4], candida overgrowth[5], colitis[6] and diverticulitis[7], and can contribute to post-natal jing deficiencies in children including ADD, ADHD and autism[8,9,10]. People with these bacterial imbalances will benefit from consuming naturally fermented foods, including kim chee, sauerkraut, yogurt, and kombucha.

The many of strains of beneficial bacteria, originally derived from our mother's milk, live and reproduce in our guts throughout our lives and play distinct and essential roles in breaking down the varying cellular structures of our foods. We will discuss the most prominent of these food types below. The tonic herbal elixirs we will discuss have not been observed to disrupt beneficial gut flora.

The Basic Nature of Foods

All vegetables, including leafy, root, stalk, and other foods that can be chewed and efficiently digested, act as carbohydrates and represent our primary fuel source. Carbohydrates include sugars, the most readily available fuel source; starches; and fats.

Sugars

There are different types of sugars. Simple monosaccharides burn very fast, creating a quick burst of false chi, and generally contain little to no additional residual nutritive value. More complex sugars, polysacharrides, are not always sweet; often we don't recognize that we are consuming a sugar when we eat them. Polysacharrides carry complex nutritive components into the bloodstream and assist in easy assimilation of agents that support immunity, adaptability, the endocrine system, the liver, and digestion. Many of the herbs I will discuss in the pages ahead contain complex polysaccharides.

Polysaccharides can be assimilated from raw food, and many remain intact after cooking or fermenting.

Starches

These nutrients are more complex carbohydrates that tend to have a locked phytochemistry. This is why we don't see many raw food recipes that include potatoes and many squashes. These foods are better cooked before consumption. Think of cooking a starch like roasting a hard corn kernel to pop it into a piece of popcorn. It is very hard for our digestive fluids to metabolize nutrients from a hard corn kernel; it must be popped. The food industry term for this popping open of the starch molecule is gelatinizing.

The most efficient way to gelatinize a starch is to roast it. The Incans roasted maca, a starchy tuber. This opens its chi. I recommend gelatinized maca in the diet. The same goes for potatoes, sweet potatoes, and yams. Starches are also broken down through fermentation, a good solution for the hard core raw foodist.

Fats

These slower-burning carbohydrates are designed by nature to "time-release" into the system in order to help the body's humors and cells maintain flexibility, blood motility, and cellular respiration. Fats support a host of bodily needs. There are two types of fats: saturated and unsaturated. Both are necessary for health. The body creates many of these fats, such as triglycerides, while some must be obtained through the diet.

Unsaturated fat molecules are generally considered healthier than saturated fats. Unsaturated fats have more than one carbon bond and fewer hydrogen molecules than saturated fats. They have a bent shape so that when agglomerated, they pile in a way that leaves spaces where other nutrients can be trapped. Fats are easily soluble—into oils. After consumption, fat molecules attach to membranes in the body be it arterial walls or other tissues—and the next time the person is out running or cutting the grass, the fat molecules break down and release their nutritive value as well as trapped nutrients into the blood stream, providing extra fuel for the body.

The liver transforms fat molecules into glycogen and triglycerides. These course in the body humors and are stored on and in tissues for future use. Triglycerides will agglomerate in the liver of a person who eats too much fat and doesn't exercise. A sedentary person will not as readily metabolize these fats back into chi. When such a person takes on a more active lifestyle, and/or begins taking herbs and foods that increase metabolism to warm the body, these fats will release fuel for metabolism and chi.

Saturated fats contain only one carbon bond and are saturated with hydrogen atoms; they cannot take on any more. Due to their simple, stick-like shape, these fats compact into denser, semisolid material. They do not allow space for other nutrients to be infused, and they form on arteries and vein walls in hard deposits that are difficult to break down. The body needs more warmth and chi to metabolize these hardened fat deposits and plaques. Saturated fats also play a role in the development of tumors. They are one of the demons created by cooking food.

This is why fats should mainly be taken whole and unsaturated. There are three types of essential fats that we must derive through our diet. They are classified according to their origins: omega–3 from animals and fish, omega–6 from foods such as avocado, and omega–9 from seeds. A good blend of these in proper ratios is suggested on a daily basis for health and for "oiling" the body. Again, most of these fats are adversely altered when heated to average cooking temperatures. Coconut oil is the only oil that appears unchanged by cooking.

Proteins

Proteins are comprised of a vast group of nutrients that are often best assimilated by heating or fermenting. Like starches, a protein molecule is fixed and has a specific use in the body. A protein molecule resembles a folded flower bud. Preparing it through heat, hydrolization, or fermentation, or using enzymes to break it down, "unfolds" the molecules, making it easier for the body to assimilate its nutrients. This is why beans and other legumes are best cooked or fermented. Black beans cooked in soup are an excellent protein source when combined with black rice. (Gut bacteria help us digest sugars and proteins in many legumes, which is where we get gas. Taking amylase and protease enzymes helps reduce this uncomfortable side effect.)

Fermenting

Fermentation with probiotic bacteria increases the available chi in foods and helps preserve their freshness. The fermenting process has also been found to reduce the negative components of isoflavones and allergens. Fermenting soybeans has been a tradition in China, Japan, and Korea for centuries. Many Asian cultures did not traditionally consume diets high in red meat, and thus, needed to have vegetarian protein sources. Because of this necessity, as well as the lack of refrigeration, they discovered the importance of fermenting foods to preserve and unlock nutrients. It's easy to ferment your own food. Virtually all carbohydrates can be fermented in your own kitchen. Strains of probiotic bacteria may be purchased in Asian supermarkets, and there are many websites that offer instructions. In my neighborhood of Upland, California, is a woman who makes personalized fermented food blends after doing a unique method of health evaluation. (You can find more information at www.coconutcow.com.)

Assets of the Raw Food Diet

Raw foods are high in inherent enzymes that prevent the secretion of excess enzymatic fluids and gastric acids from the pancreas and stomach. This makes it easier for the body to metabolize food. Other health benefits of this diet include:

- potentially more balanced blood sugar/blood pressure;
- more desirable body pH;

- less susceptibility to diseases of excess;
- more energy, focus, and adaptability;
- a cleaner body interior; and
- potentially better sleep.

Less energy (in terms of electricity, gas, etc.) is used to prepare raw food, and it is easier to clean up afterward. Most raw foods are sold with less packaging than other foods and are closer to the earth, making for a more conscientious and spiritually inspiring diet.

Potential Dangers of the Raw Food Diet

- May cause cooling of the digestive system in some people, particularly those with a highly yin constitution: most women and some men who are anemic from a vegan diet.
- May cause fluid retention, mainly in women—affecting the abdomen, hips, and/or the ankles.
- May dampen the spleen meridian (splenic system), affecting metabolism and blood physiology, including problems with the menstrual cycle (see chapter eight).

Fortunately, as we will see, the Chinese medical system has developed herbal formulas to assist the spleen meridian and chi. Let's look at a few of the assets of herbal elixirs before progressing.

- May assist chi and promote warming.
- Help the body avoid unwanted moisture retention in the middle jiao and lower extremities.
- Support distribution of chi to hands and feet and assist upright chi.
- May help the body build and maintain sufficient blood levels, thus supporting the body's capacity to carry nutrition and chi through the blood system.
- May support a normal menstrual cycle.
- Said to have adaptogenic properties.
- Contain complex polysaccharides and other nutrients not found in food.

- Support the immune system.
- Promote the body's own regulating energies against proliferation of microbes, bacteria, parasites, and fungi.

CHAPTER 7
Chi Herbs

In China, certain herbs that have been shown to cultivate and protect chi have been consumed for centuries. They are classified as tonifying chi, thereby helping support a strong constitution. Chi herbs can help increase metabolism and enhance the food-to-energy process. Chi herbs can also aid the body in transforming unwanted accumulations of water from the middle jiao. Most, if not all, of the chi herbs tonify the spleen. These herbs help ensure we maintain an adequate metabolism and protect our jing reserves. Chi herbs work to warm and activate the body's breakdown and assimilation of nutrients *without excessively stimulating the nervous system.* This is very important. They warm the middle jiao without giving one the jitters, thereby helping avoid adrenal (jing) exertion. However, herbs may be harvested before they have reached maturity or therapeutic vitality, and such poor quality or immature herbs may produce undesirable effects. The descriptions that follow include insights on how to determine the quality of chi herbs before buying them.

Quality/Purity of Chinese Herbs

Herbs cultivated in China often come from diverse regions. Some herbs may have been grown in polluted areas, in denuded soils located near industry, but I have found high-quality Chinese herbs in most herb shops. In addition to the descriptions of high-quality herbs below, I also discuss in more detail how to find high quality herbs in my online course at www.GateofLife.org.

The majority of Chinese herbs are not actually farmed but wildcrafted from forest settings. They are collected by specialists who have carried on the tradition of wildcrafting for many generations. These specialists harvest in wild forests far from human corruption and industry. One notable region is the Jilin province of Manchuria in northeastern China, which borders North Korea. Many hectares in this pristine region are protected and heavily monitored as a "biosphere" overseen by the Chinese government and the United Nations. This forested area and others, including the Huangshan Mountains in the Anhui province, are the sources of many traditional Chinese herbs. Herbs sourced from these areas will be of high quality.

Dangers do exist when sourcing Chinese herbs. Some herbs may be of low quality; they may be tainted with lead and other pollutants or other harmful agents. The color and appearance of the herbs can be good indicators of their vibrancy, and experience will soon guide you to know the best when you see it. The highest quality herbs have been sourced from small, traditional family farms in pristine regions of northern China and Korea. These farmers hand down their fields to their progeny and, by tradition, know better than to destroy their soil microbes with harmful chemicals. The Chinese are among the world's leaders in agricultural and horticultural advancements, and we in the West have learned many secrets of healthy soil from them. You may read of some of these gleanings in F. H. King's 1911 book *Farmers of Forty Centuries.*

I visited many Chinese herb farms during my first visit to China in 1985. There I saw firsthand the reverence these farmers show for the health of their soil. The Chinese have a near religious reverence for their herbs. Their use has been woven into tales of immortals and goddesses in the Chinese religions of Taoism and Buddhism. The Chinese consider their medicine to be one of the greatest gifts to humankind. From the village mothers who cook them into their family meals, to peasant collectors and farmers who have been handed down a generations-old tradition, to the sellers, I have found an impeccably high adherence to quality and conscientiousness.

My method of avoiding low-grade herbs and ensuring I buy herbs sourced from pristine forest regions is simply to buy the most expensive herbs. The price for top-grade herbs is still very affordable and well worth it. We can be assured these herbs have passed through their own checks and balances as they made their way from collector to us. Knowledgeable consumers of Chinese herbs can recognize low-grade herbs, and herb shops selling these low-quality herbs will get a bad reputation as a result. Make friends with the herbalist at your local herb shop. Ask questions about the herb sourcing. If the herbalist is not able to answer your questions about quality and such, try to find another herb shop.

You should briefly rinse herbs before decoction, as they have traveled far to get to you, and who knows what tainted fluids, air, and possible irradiation they encountered along the way.

The following are among the most renowned chi herbs.

Ginseng

Ginseng *(see below for various varieties)* is a premier chi herb. Good ginseng is considered an adaptogen. It can strengthen our basic capacity to adjust, both mentally and physically, to changes in circumstance or environment. Ginseng that is at least seven years old contains multidimensional nutrients, such as ginsenosides, complex polysaccharides that are highly empowering, immune modulating antioxidants. Such nutrients increase our physical and emotional endurance and adaptability.

The historical documentation of ginseng in Asia is immense and illustrious. The Chinese have always held ginseng in the highest esteem for its power-enhancing qualities. In the United States, this precious herb is not fully understood, even though it was consumed by the first Americans and European newcomers since Colonial days. Ginseng must be allowed to mature before it is harvested; otherwise, its phytochemistry will not be balanced. Prematurely harvested ginseng that is phytochemically immature will produce a "unidirectional" stimulating effect similar to the alkaloids in roasted coffee. Far too many Western herbal products appear to contain these immature ginsengs, as evidenced by a widespread incidence of the reported side effect of feeling jittery. Making products with immature ginseng is a good example of Western industry's impatience with allowing plants to properly mature before harvesting.

There are many varieties of ginseng: Korean ginseng *(hong sam)* is very stimulating and warming, or yang; American ginseng *(Panax quinquefolius)* is more depth recharging, or yin; Chinese ginseng *(Panax ginseng)* is generally processed to be slightly warming. Processed Chinese ginseng will have a dark red root, whereas unprocessed Chinese ginseng is pale brown. For simplicity's sake, ginseng in general is classified as supporting chi.

Depending on the ginseng plant's origin and on how the roots are processed, this herb's potential therapeutic properties can cover a wide range, from calming and restoring to highly invigorating. For instance, traditional practices for processing ginseng in Korea involve steaming the herb with very yang herbs, such as aconite, in order to help the ginseng produce a warming effect on the consumer. This process has been practiced there for thousands of years to help people adapt to the harshly cold winters in this northern longitude (near Siberia). If Westerners take ginseng without knowing it is Korean ginseng, they may be over-stimulated from the yang properties in this variety of the herb and then form an ill-conceived opinion about the overall effects of ginseng. Such energy and yang-enhancing processes were never applied to American ginseng, and by the time Colonial settlers recognized its value, the Chinese were the first large-scale customers for our domestic ginseng. They appreciate it particularly for its calming yin properties.

Native American peoples were well aware of ginseng's health-enhancing properties. The herb played a role in early U.S. history. The British ship that spurred the Boston Tea Party was carrying a load of black tea from China intended to be traded for ginseng. If the raid by American Colonists, who infamously dumped the tea into the harbor in protest of the taxes levied by the British, had taken place a few hours later, the event would have been known as the "Boston Ginseng Party" in our history books. Daniel Boone, of early pioneering fame, was a ginseng poacher. He made his living searching for the plants in Kentucky, filling barges with them, and shipping them to the north for export to China. Unfortunately, he was not a very successful businessman because he consistently overfilled his barges with ginseng, causing them to sink.

Here's what one Colonel Byrd had to say about ginseng sometime in the late 1800s:

Though practice will soon make a man of tolerable Vigour an able footman, yet, as a help to bear fatigue I us'd to chew the root of Ginseng as I walk't along. This Kept up my spirits and made me trip away as nimbly in my half jack-boots as younger men cou'd in their shoes. This plant is in high esteem in China, where it sells for its weight in silver . . . Its virtues are, that it gives an uncommon warmth and vigour to the blood, and frisks the spirits, beyond any other cordial. It cheers the heart . . . helps the memory and would quicken even Helvetian dullness. 'Tis friendly to the lungs, much more than scolding itself. . . . And what is more, it will even make old age amiable, by rendering it lively, cheerful, and good humour'd.[11]

Wild ginsengs are considered far superior in quality to cultivated or semicultivated plants. Cultivated ginsengs are usually farm grown and often harvested at an early stage. Semicultivated ginsengs are plants that were discovered in the wild but deemed too young for harvesting. The discoverer provided irrigation, soil fortification, and protection from predator animals until the plants were ready for harvest. Semiwild, semicultivated ginsengs are easy to spot at an herb bazaar. The top half will generally have a rougher topography, with deep, dark lines or striations; this is the part of the herb that developed in the wild. The bottom area will be lighter and generally clear of striations. This section represents the growth of the ginseng root after someone made its life easier with water and TLC. The cultivated part will have less therapeutic value than the deeply striated wild part because fewer inherent nutrients were compacted in the marrow of the cultivated part and there was not as much need to develop defenses against the ravages of nature.

A ginseng root will not develop the adaptogenic properties that make it valuable for our consumption until it is about eight years old. Before this time, the plant is dominated by yang growth hormones. Ginseng consumed during this stage will produce an effect similar to that of coffee. Not realizing the importance of the plant's age, Americans often purchase immature ginseng products. Many buyers on the herb market will pay low prices for these herbs, promoting a policy where growers find it profitable to harvest ginseng before it matures.

Nature's wisdom keeps ginseng from developing its therapeutic potential earlier in order to allow a process of natural selection to take place. In its early stages, ginseng is a plant like any other. Foraging animals, crowding, and bad weather conditions can weed out all but the strongest plants. If ginseng had its powerful properties from the beginning, it would have crowded out most other plant forms by now.

Once the ginseng plants that survive this initial vulnerable period reach their eighth year, they seem to undergo a genealogic upgrading, developing the capacity to withstand severe drought or flood, extremes of cold and hot, and other natural challenges. They begin to produce natural antibiotic properties that help to fend off the damage of infections inflicted by foraging critters. The plant is now mature enough that when the sun shines on its leaves, power flows back down into the marrow of the root, helping it to develop yin properties deep in the root core. Over time, the root will develop its adaptogenic or "dual-directional" properties. As the root further ages, it will accumulate additional yin properties in the marrow and yang energy at the surface, thus fostering balance and adaptability. As a ginseng root ages beyond ten or fifteen years, it seems to take on the appearance of an aged and wizened human; this is why the Chinese call ginseng "man root." Legend has it that mature ginseng actually starts to develop the capacity to invoke *wisdom* in the consumer. This can explain why wild, old ginseng roots can fetch such high prices at markets in China. A fifty-year-old wild ginseng root can sell for $20,000.

However, because they are so prized, wild ginseng roots are almost impossible to find in China nowadays. This is why they command such a lofty price. Many ginseng hunters lose their lives every year trying to scale high cliffs while searching for ginseng in the crags. This kind of wild ginseng is especially soughtafter, as the plants found growing in the most inhospitable regions are thought to contain the highest concentrations of power by virtue of enduring such difficult living conditions.

Ginseng plants are thought to contain a subtle, barely detectable luminescence, which some hunters cultivate the ability to see on dark moonless nights. Because ginseng plants are said to "hide" in inaccessible places, they may not be noticeable during the day. Ginseng hunters will go out on dark nights with bow and arrow. When they see the luminescence of a ginseng plant that is hiding in an inaccessible area, they will shoot a flagged arrow in the direction of the ginseng, return to the vicinity in the morning, find the arrow, and discover the ginseng nearby.

When purchasing ginseng, one should make the effort to learn the origins of the plant's species and its general "atmospheric energy" (yin/yang and heating/cooling properties) before consuming it. Good resource books about ginseng include Ron Teeguarden's *The Ancient Wisdom of the Chinese Tonic Herbs* and Michael Tierra's *The Way of Chinese Herbs.*[12] Going to Chinese herb shops and looking at ginseng can prove insightful. But beware, some high-priced, purportedly old ginsengs may be fake. Called "art ginseng," they may be merely young, immature roots that have had striations cut into them with sharp blades and dirt rubbed into the recesses, as well as extra roots craftily glued onto their sides and extra nodes attached to the stems, giving them the appearance of older ginseng roots. A trained eye with a good magnifying glass can detect these fake ginsengs.

*No contraindications are noted for high-quality ginseng. The immature, cheap stuff may cause nervousness. Korean ginseng is contraindicated for those with hypertension, high blood pressure, and a yang constitution. Chinese and American varieties are extremely safe.

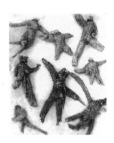

Ginseng men

Wild Chinese ginseng. Note the many nodules on the stem, indicating age.

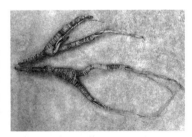

Codonopsis

Codonopsis *(dang shen)* is an herb similar to ginseng but milder in its energies. A great chi tonic, it can be used when individuals have weak spleen chi (insufficient digestion, edema in the abdominal area, loose stool, prolapse of organs in the middle-lower jiao) but prefer or need something

45

milder than ginseng, which can at times be too potent for some. Codonopsis is substituted in many formulas that once contained ginseng because in some cases it was found to work better. The primary example of this is a formula called ginseng and astragalus, the most commonly used spleen chi formula. It actually contains codonopsis instead of ginseng. The story goes that during a period of the great Chinese dynasties, the ginseng and astragalus formula was used extensively for many conditions, including immune fortifying. The plant became scarce due to heavy consumption, and then a period of drought made it even scarcer. The available ginseng was reserved for the emperor's family. Herbalists at that time knew the codonopsis rhizome had properties and effects similar to ginseng but not as powerful. For the general populace, codonopsis was substituted for ginseng, and soon the common folks were having better results with the revised formula than the ruling class was with the original.

There is another lesson here: certain combinations of herbs will bring out more dominant or efficacious qualities that do not manifest when the herbs are taken alone or in other combinations. This is the true sophistication of the Chinese system; 4,000 odd years of experimentation has yielded extremely refined formula. *Codonopsis* was permanently substituted and became the general "emperor" herb, or dominant factor of this formula, instead of ginseng, even though it is milder in its overall effects as an isolated herb. Interestingly, the name "ginseng and astragalus formula" remained the same because by that time the formula had become a well-known commodity in China. It is similar to how a company might modify the ingredients in a popular cereal brand but still call it by the original name.

Codonopsis should be flexible and chewy. It should be a tan color and should not be pock-marked with black spots.

*Contraindications: none listed, very safe.

White Atractylodes

White Atractylodes (*bai zhu*) is my favorite spleen chi herb. Rather an unsung hero of the tonic herb hierarchy, it is the most effective herb for drying moisture from the middle jiao and activating the spleen. This herb helps turn up the fire under the stomach and wrest chi from the food we've eaten. White atractylodes is commonly found in formulas designed for counteracting accumulated dampness in the stomach/spleen area and is highly regarded in Chinese medicine. The herb is especially important for those who choose to eat high proportions of living, uncooked food in their diet. Though Chinese medical authorities do not recommend eating much raw food, I have determined in my work that herbal teas containing white atractylodes may act as tonics for spleen chi when taken *along with* raw foods, possibly helping prevent unwanted moisture accumulation. I am hoping to initiate a paradigm shift in Chinese thinking about raw food and spleen chi by recommending spleen chi teas as a dietary component taken along with foods known to be cooling in nature.

White atractylodes should be off-white to yellow with gold and orange speckles. Most all white atractylodes on the market is of similar quality.

*Contraindications: do not use excessively when dehydrated.

Poria

Poria *(fu ling)* is usually combined with white atractylodes in formulas for the spleen, blood, and removal of moisture. Poria is famed by Chinese women as an excellent aid in the maintenance of a good figure. It is said to help transform dampness into chi. Poria helps remove extra dampness while white atractylodes warms the digestion (I will discuss poria further in chapter eight).

*Contraindications: none listed, very safe.

Aged Citrus Peel

Aged citrus peel *(chen pi)* warms the middle jiao, regulates chi, improves the function of the spleen, and relieves stagnant chi in the stomach, such as abdominal distention, bloating, and loose stool. It is said to help relieve nausea and vomiting. Citrus peel dries dampness and transforms phlegm. It's also helpful for damp phlegm in the lung. While citrus peel is not considered a tonic herb, it works well as an adjunct in formulas to assist in the breakup of chi stagnation.

*Contraindications: this is not a tonic herb and is only used as a warming adjunct in spleen chi formulas.

Immature Citrus Fruit

Immature citrus fruit *(qing pi)* is said to have "thermogenic" action in the body, that is, it helps warm the insides to a point where we can begin to break down fats and utilize them for energy. Remember that fats are carbohydrate storage houses, so any whole fat molecule that is metabolized into the bloodstream will also release other nutrients at the same time, allowing the body to derive more materials for combustion of chi energy. Immature citrus fruit is the new herb of choice for weight loss.

Cinnamon Twig

Cinnamon twig *(gui zhi)* warms the middle jiao and helps break up chi stagnation with stimulating effects. Cinnamon twig is very helpful in any dieter's formula and contains unique properties to help manage weight and stimulate chi. The pieces are usually short and cyndrical in shape and should have the strong aroma of cinnamon.

Coix

Coix *(yi yi ren)* is a grain similar to barley in both appearance and effect. Coix warms and nurtures digestion and assists in the passage of the food bolus through the duodenum and small intestine. Coix pieces resemble whole barley and should be white in color.

Jujube Date

Jujube date *(hong zao)* is a red date that is perhaps more commonly known in the West than many other Chinese herbs. A famed spleen chi herb, red jujube invigorates and revitalizes the general metabolism. Jujube has a general warming effect on the middle jiao, the digestive tract. It helps increase appetite and relieve loose stool. Jujube nourishes the blood and calms the spirit. As Dan Bensky said, it is supportive "for wan appearance, irritability and emotional lability due to restless organ disorder."[13] A wonderful-tasting smoked jujube date is also sometimes used, and it is thought to be more yang than the red jujube. The black smoked jujube is not used as much because it does not remain fresh in a sealed, airtight bag; it can become moldy and therefore is not relied upon for storage in Chinese herb shops. The smaller jujube dates are better, the best ones being about the size of a large almond. They come with or without the seed and should be torn or cut in half before decocting.

*Contraindications: avoid jujube when there is excess phlegm in the body along with abdominal bloating, food retention, and/or parasites.

Licorice Root

Licorice root *(gan cao)* is a very important herb. It moderates the characteristics of other herbs it is combined with, harmonizing hot and cold herbs. It also mitigates the potential side effects of some herbs. This versatile root has shown a myriad of benefits in recent Western studies. I use it mainly in spleen chi formulas for men and in detox formulas, as it is an excellent and mild broad-spectrum blood cleanser. An excellent lung tonic for coughs and wheezing, it is considered a neutral herb and thus may be used for either hot, dry or cold, damp conditions in the lungs. Licorice clears heat in the body and controls spasms, alleviating pain[14.]

Caution: Excess consumption of licorice root has been linked to a rise in blood pressure in some individuals. Those who are on blood pressure medication may wish to substitute jujube date in this formula. A deglycerized form of licorice root extract may be attained from pharmacies. It is said that high-quality licorice root must be grown for more than two years before harvesting. This high-quality licorice root may have a lower propensity to adversely affect blood pressure. Ask the herbalists at your local Chinese herb shop for "two-year licorice." (For a further discourse on licorice, refer to www.umm.edu/altmed/articles/licorice-000262.htm.)

Harmonizing Chi

Jujube date and licorice root are the two most commonly used herbs in the Chinese *Materia medica.* The Chinese say that the inclusion of one or both of these herbs brings all the myriad of herbs in the formula into harmony, so that the various therapeutic actions of the herbal blend are melded into unity of purpose and then harmonized within the body. Jujube date and licorice root are essential herbs in any true Chinese herbal formula. Their absence may indicate that the formula was designed by an inexperienced herbalist. These two herbs in particular harmonize spleen chi and are therefore included in this section, yet they are also used to harmonize formulas designed to tonify other organ meridians, bodily, and spiritual energies.

The herbs we have discussed represent a small minority of herbs in the Chinese *Materia medica*, yet every formula that is used to tonify chi will contain one or more of these herbs in varying quantities. The combinations and ratios of the herbs will help produce selective effects on the regulation of chi in the body.

JUJUBE DATE (RED) *(hong zao)*

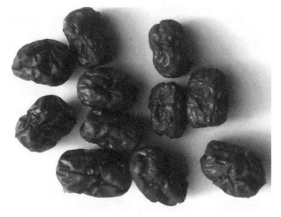

"Harmonizer" in herbal formulas, chi

CODONOPSIS *(dang shen)*

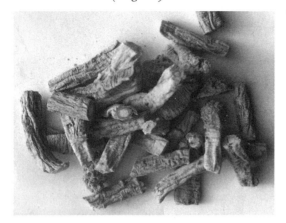

"Ginseng for Women"

WHITE ATRACTYLODES *(bai zhu)*

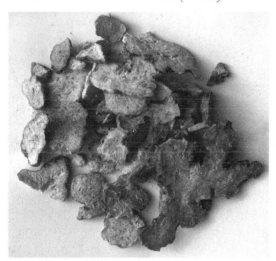

Warms the middle jiao

PORIA *(fu ling)*

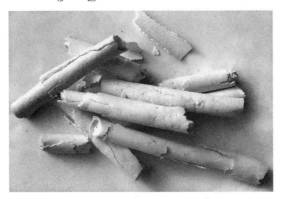

Steams off dampness

LICORICE ROOT *(gan cao)*

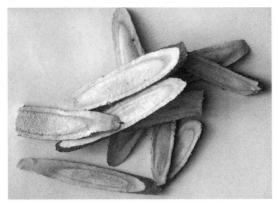

Another harmonizer
and blood cleanser

Tea formulations containing herbs that warm the middle jiao and activate spleen chi can be very effective when taken along with diets high in raw foods. The spleen chi tea outlined below is my recommendation to help warm the middle in order to enhance digestion and eliminate moistness and water retention, which can be a particularly problematic issue for many women, as I will discuss in chapter eight.

A Chi Elixir

In I gallon water,

Codonopsis *(dang shen):* 2–3 ounces or I large handful *or*
    Chinese ginseng *(Panax):* I ounce or small handful*
White Atractylodes *(bai zhu):* 2–3 ounces or I large handful
Rehmannia, prepared *(shu di huang):* 3 ounces or I handful
Poria *(fu ling):* 2–3 ounces or I large handful (8–I0 pieces if tubular)
Astragalus *(huang qi):* I–2 ounces or I large handful
Jujube date† *(da zao):* 2–3 ounces or I large handful

*Break or crush ginseng into small bits.
† Tear or cut jujube date in half before decocting.

For full cooking/decocting instructions, see the appendix.

Adaptogens for Chi

The majority of tonic herbs in the Chinese herbal system contain properties that are defined as adaptogenic. These herbs have been found over centuries of use to balance the body's energies through a dual-directional benefit on the forces of yin and yang. This is one of the major criteria by which they attain their elite status as tonic herbs. Adaptogenic herbs support a balanced central nervous system and immune system and help to regulate the circadian rhythms.

Research conducted in the 1940s by Russian doctors Lazarov and Brekhman[15] on the herbs rhodiola and Eleutherococcus (formerly Siberian ginseng) determined that these herbs can help balance the sympathetic and parasympathetic subcomponents of the central nervous system. Rhodiola and eleutherococcus can lessen stress, inflammatory symptoms, and muscular constriction. These herbs provide adaptogenic support for the immune system, helping balance potential immune-related inflammation and insufficient immune response. The research also found that adaptogenic herbs can be taken daily to support our day/night, work/relax rhythms. When taken in the morning, these herbs can help stimulate the body into action, and if taken in the evening, they can help the body

53

begin to wind down for the night. Regular use of adaptogenic herbs can help reduce symptoms of PMS and menopause.[16] Adaptogenic herbs include rhodiola (rosea and crenulata), eleutherococcus, ginseng (*Panax*), astragalus (*huang chi*) and lycium (*goji*).

Adaptogenic Chi Elixir

Astragalus *(huang chi):* 2–3 ounces or 1 large handful

Rhodiola *(rosea or crenulata):* ¼ teaspoon powdered extract

Eleutherococcus (formerly called Siberian ginseng): 2–3 ounces or 1 handful

Lycium *(goji):* 2–3 ounces or 1 handful

Licorice root *(gan cao):* 1 ounce or 1 small handful

See appendix for cooking instructions.

CHAPTER 8
Women: Yin and Blood

In general, women have a yin constitution. This means that they take in and absorb life's essences, and they store this energy as jing. Life requires this of women because they are the bringers of new life, which requires an extra storehouse of jing energy to draw upon from conception through the child's rearing into young adulthood. To accumulate the extra energy reserves needed for conceiving, birthing, and raising children, women need to convert more vital chiinto jing; thus, the female energy is *receptive*—it is yin.

Yin is best represented by water, a fluid that can absorb other essences and materials and distribute and hold them in suspension. Some women are more yin than others, but most are generally said to be ruled by yin. The Chinese classify raw foods as yin due to their cool and watery nature. The reason doctors of traditional Chinese medicine discourage a highly raw diet is that people with yin constitutions will become overly watery if they consume too many yin foods.

Many women are susceptible to excess moisture retention, edema, and bloating. These accumulations are usually noticed in the hips and abdomen. Women need chi to stimulate warmth in the middle and lower jiaos (reproductive organs/glands and excretory organs). Chi energy helps steam off the unwanted moisture and transform it into chi. It is best for women to maintain good nutritive sources of chi as well as practice phranic deep breathing exercises, so that moisture is transformed into energy and does not have time to collect. Should this watery distention occur, a woman will by then probably have a dampened spleen, which can lead to more problems with general energy, metabolism, and blood building—including anomalies with the menstrual cycle. Chi is carried in the blood, and so the Chinese say that women are governed by blood and blood is the carrier of chi.

Most of my female clients report having menstrual irregularities. I give them herbs to build blood and tonify chi, which seems to help significantly. Years of seeing their improvements in general energy, mood, and moon cycle regularity led me to the conclusions I am writing about in this book. I believe with proper chi in women's diets, and with correct breathing, we can see much better overall health of body, mind, and the reproductive cycle. Let's first look at what can lead to problems.

Due to a chi-less diet derived from the available foodstuffs on grocery store shelves, many young girls have irregular menstrual cycles. Most commonly, they experience excessive menstrual bleeding over longer periods. This is because their blood isn't infused with enough chi. Chi vitalizes the blood to flow upright to the hands, feet, head, and back around. Keeping the chi upright helps prevent the downward trickling of blood.

Blood that lacks sufficient chi will be darker, thicker, and sluggish, with possible accumulations of clots and masses. These can build up in the lower jiao, where chi stagnation most readily occurs in the presence of edema. With insufficient upright chi, the blood will trickle downward and accumulate in the abdomen, in and possibly around the uterus. This trickling occurs mainly in the ovular stage of the moon cycle, which is natural because the blood is intended to create a lining for a placenta.

At ovulation, during mid-month, the body should be warmed by about one degree via an infusion of progesterone into the blood stream, reinstating upright chi and ceasing the downward trickling of blood into the uterine cavity. With good chi from the diet and healthily regulated hormone synthesis, the menstrual period should be regular, light, and easy. But some young women who starve themselves on rice crackers in order to look like the models on TV breathe shallowly so as not to extend their belly and pelvis. They also likely take birth control. All of these actions deprive women of chi, phrana, and hormonal balance/support. Their blood has insufficient chi. It trickles downward, leaving their hands and feet cold and resulting in general lethargy. They will experience cramping and excessive bleeding during their menstrual periods, and their blood will be thick and dark.

This Leads to Damp Spleen

Next comes the accumulation of moisture in the middle and lower jiao. Blood, being the carrier of chi, is not bringing nutritive essences to the body, and the boiler room of the body, the spleen/pancreas does not receive enough fuel. The fire of life is at low flame. The spleen doesn't have enough octane to wrest the iron and other nutrients from ingested foods, and new iron ions are not being freed to insert into the blood. When blood passing through the spleen is not picking up necessary chi as iron, the blood lacks its upright chi potential, which leads to cold hands and feet. Since the middle jiao is not warm enough, moisture from the foods these women eat and the liquids they drink cannot be adequately steamed off into chi. Moisture accumulates around the middle jiao. When this cold

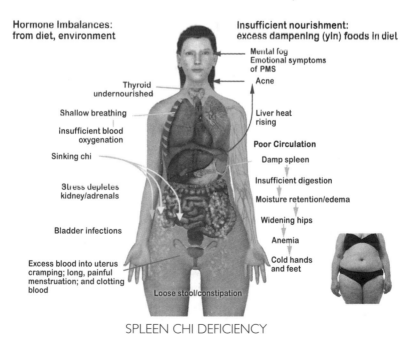

Hormone Imbalances:
from diet, environment

Insufficient nourishment:
excess dampening (yin) foods in diet

Mental fog
Emotional symptoms
of PMS

Acne

Thyroid
undernourished

Shallow breathing

Liver heat
rising

Insufficient blood
oxygenation

Poor Circulation

Sinking chi

Damp spleen

Insufficient digestion

Stress depletes
kidney/adrenals

Moisture retention/edema

Widening hips

Bladder infections

Anemia

Excess blood into uterus
cramping; long, painful
menstruation; and clotting
blood

Cold hands
and feet

Loose stool/constipation

SPLEEN CHI DEFICIENCY

accumulation occurs, we need to take measures to warm the middle jiao. The raw food diet does not necessarily help, as it is considered a yin and cooling diet. This is exactly why the Chinese acupuncturists discourage it. Here we will examine an illustration (on page 57) that depicts the many common metabolic, hormonal, and emotional problems that many women experience to differing degrees, including the confounding bloating from accumulations of moisture around the middle jiao.

Yet this is also where I made my breakthrough. There are Chinese herbs that support spleen chi and help remove dampness and warm the middle jiao. We discussed these herbs—white atractylodes, poria, codonopsis, jujube, cinnamon twig, citrus peel, and coix—in the previous chapter.

Certain herbs are also traditionally used to help build blood. This is another way in which the Chinese herbal elixirs I describe in this book can be of immense value.

Building Blood

Blood carries chi throughout the body. It must be vitalized and plentiful. This is why women are governed by blood, as contrasted with men, who don't have such issues since they don't lose blood every month.

Again, the Chinese have gifted humanity with developments and discoveries in blood maintenance. This is because the Chinese were never heavy eaters of red meat. Over the centuries, they witnessed women's fertility cycles and recognized that they needed supplements of herbs and foods that helped build blood. They sought foods high in iron and zinc, and they found herbs that appeared to help build and maintain adequate ratios of blood for health.

The primary herb for building blood is *dang gui*. Dang gui is found in herbal formulas for anemia and sluggish chi. The herb is said to increase estrogen, but studies by Subhuti Dharmananda, a leader in Chinese herbology, reveal that dang gui subtly supports estrone, one of the good estrogens, maintaining it in ratios far under any dangerous levels.[17] As a folk technique in China, menstruating women steam dang gui with spinach for meals during the ovular (early) stage of the monthly fertility cycle.

The Chinese also realized that blood and chi need to be vitalized, and the movement of blood needs to be promoted. They found herbs to move blood and chi, thereby helping prevent chi stagnation, particularly during the menstrual period. The most notable of these is white peony root *(bai shao)*. White peony root helps break up chi stagnation and is indispensable in herbal elixirs and formulas for assisting the free flow of chi, from muscle strain to menstrual cramping.

Another herb that supports and fortifies blood is ligusticum *(gao ben)*. Ligusticum enriches the blood. It is a relative of celery and is only cooked for short periods (see the appendix for tea preparation).

The herb rehmannia glutinosa *(shu di huang)* is a wonderful blood vitalizer that helps resonate chi to the kidney jing. Rehmannia is a famed all-round tonic said to be "the kidney's own food." When included in chi formulas, this herb broadens the benefits of the long-term accumulated energy of the body's creative and procreative forces.

These four herbs constitute a basic blood formula the Chinese simply call "Four Things Combination." This combination also represents a blood-building entity in larger formulas and may be combined with the herbs for tonifying spleen chi. Such combinations are very beneficial for women.

DANG GUI (lat. *Angelica sinensis*)

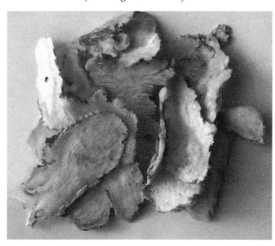

Build blood

LIGUSTICUM (*gao ben*)

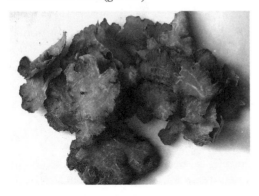

Nourish blood and heart

WHITE PEONY ROOT (*bai shao*)

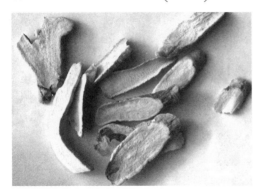

Break up chi stagnation

REHMANNIA GLUTINOSA (*shu di huang*)

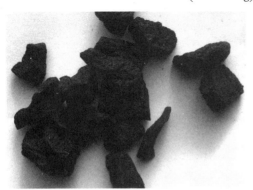

Nourish jing and fortify blood

SCHIZANDRA (*wu wei zi*)

The "Five Tastes herb"

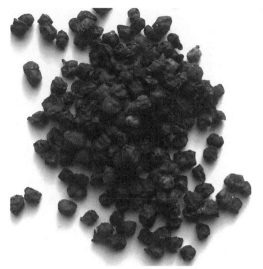

A Women's Herbal Elixir for Blood and Chi

Build blood *(dang gui)*, move and vitalize blood (white peony root), tonify kidney yin and enhance blood (prepared rehmannia), tonify spleen, warm the middle jiao (white atractylodes), transform dampness, and relieve bloating (poria) due to edema and fluid retention.

Dang gui *(Angelica sinensis):* 1 ounce or ½ handful

White peony *(bai shao):* 2–3 ounces or 1 large handful

Rehmannia, prepared *(shu di huang):* 3 ounces or 1 handful

White Atractylodes *(bai zhu):* 2–3 ounces or 1 handful

Poria *(fu ling):* 2 ounces or 1 handful (8–10 pieces if tubular)

Ligusticum* *(gao ben):* 1 ounce or 1 handful

Jujube date† *(da zao):* 2 ounces

Schizandra‡ *(wu wei zi):* 1 ounce

*Add Ligusticum during the last five minutes of cooking.

†Tear or cut jujube date in half before cooking.

‡Add schizandra berries during the last three minutes of cooking.

Detailed cooking/preparation instructions are in the appendix.

As mentioned earlier, there are herbs in the Chinese Pharmacopoeia that are said to support hormones, particularly progesterone. Progesterone helps warm the body when it is infused into the blood at ovulation. Women can support progesterone in regulating estrogen buildup in the bloodstream and body. Younger menstruating women (under ideal circumstances) produce a flood of progesterone into the bloodstream at ovulation, but as women age and fewer eggs are released from the ovaries during mid-month, it is helpful to supplement progesterone in the form of natural creams and herbal teas.

The Chinese have traditionally used a wild yam to assist in the production of progesterone. This yam, called *dioscorea,* is high in diosgenins, precursors to progesterone. Taking dioscorea in tea can help women with general hormone regulation, although Dr. John Lee and others claim that the dioscorea yam must be processed in a priority method to make it useful as a progesterone supporter. Dr. Lee pioneered the use of natural progesterone creams made from this wild yam. Asian women merely drink it in herbal teas.

I believe dioscorea indirectly benefits chi via endocrine support in bodily invigoration.

DIOSCOREA (*shan yao*)

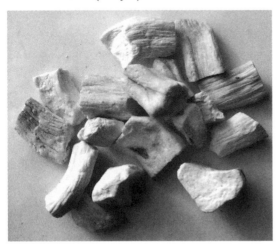

An Elixir for Assisting Female Hormone Balance

Dioscorea provides diosgenins, a phyto-progesterone source. Pain and menstrual cramping can be relieved by white peony root. Ligusticum vitalizes the blood and heart. Tribulus is tonic to the reproductive chi in both sexes.

> **Dioscorea** *(shan yao):* 2–3 ounces or 1 large handful
>
> **Dang gui** *(Angelica sinensis):* 1 ounce or ½ handful
>
> **White peony root** *(bai shao):* 2–3 ounces or 1 large handful
>
> **Rehmannia, prepared** *(shu di huang):* 3 ounces or 1 handful
>
> **Tribulus** *(bai ji li):* 1–2 ounces or 1 handful
>
> **Lycium** *(go ji ze):* 1–2 ounces or 1 handful
>
> **Jujube date*** *(hong zao):* 2–3 ounces or 1 handful
>
> **Ligusticum†** *(gao ben):* 1 ounce or ½ handful
>
> **Schizandra‡** *(wu wei zi):* 1 ounce

* Tear or cut jujube date in half before cooking.

† Add ligusticum during the last five minutes of cooking.

‡ Add schizandra during the last three minutes of cooking.

For cooking/preparation instructions, see the appendix.

Supporting Chi and Jing

We are very fortunate that for centuries the Chinese have documented the positive benefits of herbs that can be used in conjunction to nourish both chi and jing simultaneously. For women, chi and jing should be nourished together because women need more chi stored as jing in order to propagate future life as well as navigate their later years with vitality and adaptability. The more a woman has sourced sufficient chi and has stored it in the well-house of jing, the easier her transformations at mid-life will be. Such fortunate women may manage stress more easily and enter a new level of power, while also retaining their femininity. In order for women to feel true vitality, the reproductive forces and associated glands/organs must be nourished and maintained. The following is a basic standard formula I give to almost all women. This formula includes the herb ho shou wu *(Polygonum multiflorum)*, which is famed in China as a youth restoring herb—a direct fortifier of jing.

HO SHO WU *(Polygonum multiflorum)*

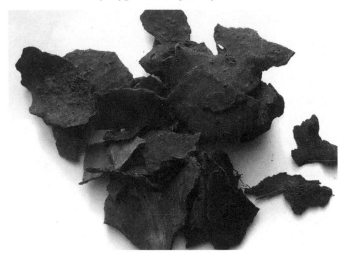

An Elixir for Assisting Female Chi and Jing

Ho shou wu is a famous anti-aging herb associated with fertility and youth. It helps fight the ravages of stress.

> **Ho shou wu** *(Polygonum multiflorum):* 4 ounces or 1 large handful
> **Rehmannia, prepared** *(shu di huang):* 3 ounces or 1 handful
> **White Atractylodes** *(bai zhu):* 3 ounces or 1 large handful
> **Poria** *(fu ling):* 3 ounces or 1 handful
> **Dioscorea** *(shan yao):* 2–3 ounces or 1 large handful
> **Dang gui** *(Angelica sinensis):* 1 ounce or ½ handful
> **Jujube date*** *(hong zao):* 2–3 ounces or 1 handful
> **Schizandra†** *(wu wei zi):* 1 ounce

* Tear or cut jujube date in half before cooking.
† Add schizandra during the last three minutes of cooking.

For cooking/preparation instructions, see the appendix.

Beautiful Chi

We cannot leave the discussion without devoting a moment to women's beauty. Where chi flows, beauty follows. Chi brings nutrients to the capillaries and ensures energy will not stagnate and erupt as inflammation. A free flow of chi helps ensure our body's largest organ gets nutritional support for elasticity and immune support in order to protect us from airborne and waterborne carcinogens as well as agents that cause free radicals.

The Chinese believe the body's exterior is protected by a branch of the immune system they call the *wei chi*. This branch is found just below the surface of the skin and helps neutralize harmful agents that could penetrate the skin or be absorbed. Upright chi and wei chi are interdependent. Chi must flow throughout the body evenly and sufficiently so that therapeutic agents may be distributed to the skin. In true health, we look to the interior, but the exterior is a barometer of our overall health, so we want the skin to reflect the radiant beauty we seek to maintain inside. When chi is flowing throughout the body's internal organs and energy is well distributed, when the body's warm chi is felt at the extremities, this will be reflected as a glowing radiance.

Once again, the Chinese knew this, and they found herbs that nourish the skin and the wei chi. The most notable herb for supporting upright chi is astragalus *(huang chi)*. This root is indisputably one of the top tonics in Chinese herbology. It enjoys a long history of beneficial use in China with no record of side effects. Astragalus is a major immune-supporting herb that helps distribute healthy immune energy to the extremities and to the subdermal layers of the skin.

Another famed herb for beauty is schizandra. Schizandra is the only herb in existence that is said to tonify all five organ meridians. In addition to assisting chi and metabolism, schizandra enjoys an illustrious position as a top beauty herb. This is because, as a harmonizer of the five organ meridians, it brings the body's energetic forces into harmony and thereby promotes a cheerful attitude and a peaceful countenance. It is said that if women take schizandra for ninety days, they will be bestowed with a perpetual smile. Schizandra is the famed beauty herb used by the goddess Quan Yin.

Pearl (margarita) is the most popular beauty herb in the world. Mucopolysacharrides in pearl have collagen-like properties and support the moisture-retaining capacity of skin cells. When skin cells retain moisture, they are less likely to develop wrinkles.

When combined with chi herbs, these three herbs can assist in the preservation of women's beauty.

A Beauty Elixir

Pearl *(Margarita):* ¼ teaspoon powder

Astragalus *(huang chi):* 2 ounces or one handful

Lycium *(goji):* 2–3 ounces or 2 handfuls

Ho shou wu *(Polygonum multiflorum):* 2–3 ounces or two handfuls

Dang gui *(Angelica sinensis):* I ounce or ½ handful

Jujube date* *(da zao):* 2–3 ounces or I handful

Schizandra† *(wu wei zi):* I ounce

* Tear or cut jujube dates in half before cooking.
† Add schizandra during the last three minutes of cooking.

For cooking/preparation instructions, refer to the appendix.

CHAPTER 9
Men: Yang and Chi

While women are governed by blood, men are generally governed by chi. This means that men must quickly assimilate chi from food and air so that they have the energy they need for their daily physical activities. Being yang by nature, most men expend their energy, and their energy stores must be supplemented accordingly. Being yin in nature, women accumulate, store, and hold chi energies as jing to build new blood, nourish their babies, and later in life, to support themselves after menopause. Men's yang is called upon to build the house or carve out the cave in which the women will bear and nurture the family's children. The man who has built a well fortified castle will also derive benefits from the nurturing/giving essences of the female, and the house will be well constructed, well defended, and full of the nurturing energies of love.

Men in the raw food community have lean, stringy muscles, as opposed to women, who may accumulate yin fluids and possibly experience moisture retention. Men should strive to consume slow-burning foods, such as whole unsaturated fats, cooked starches, and proteins, as these provide timed-released energy. Men also benefit greatly from a raw food diet, as raw foods can help cool and moisten their yang energy, which helps to protect the heart and adrenals.

Foods for Men

Here is a partial list of foods that help men fortify chi and yang, as well as those that support alkalinity and yin.

Quinoa	Miso soup
Amaranth (ground)	Barley
Chia (ground)	Oatmeal
Lentil soup	Brassica vegetables
Brown and black rice	All raw fruit and berries
Black beans	All raw, green, leafy vegetables
Plantains	All root vegetables
Yucca	Ginger
Sweet potatoes	Turmeric
Squash	

Herbs for Men

ASTRAGALUS *(huang chi)* is a major supporter of upright chi, wei chi, and general immunity and adaptability. This is one of the world's great tonic herbs for general health.

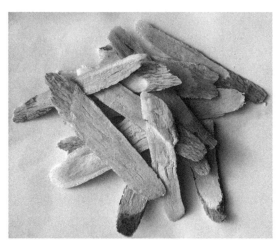

Supporting upright chi and wei chi; general immunity; adaptogen

EUCOMMIA BARK *(du zhong)* looks like snake skin and has a ligament-like latex in its structure. Eucommia bark helps support bone density and is a yang jing herb.

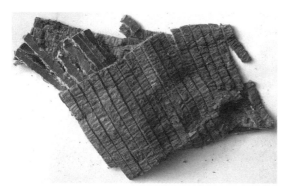

Bone, tendon, ligament, yang jing

MORINDA *(ba ji tian)* is a mildly yang herb, the root of the noni plant.

Yang jing

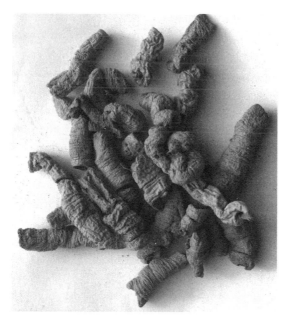

TRIBULUS *(Bulgarus terrestris, so named for its origin in Bulgaria)* is also a powerful herb for warming the yang, thereby assisting chi and jing. This "athlete's herb" is great for men and women and is said to fortify the reproductive forces in both sexes.

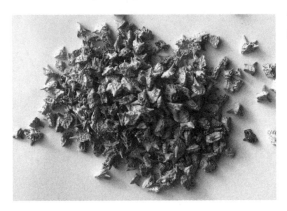

Yang jing; sexual and athletic endurance

Being yang in nature, men burn energy very fast. Because they can become yin deficient men need to drink lots of pure spring water and supplement with herbs that tonify yin, including ophiopogon, fritillaria, asparagus root, ligustrum, and schizandra. Any variation of these may be added into tea formulas for tonifying chi and yang. These herbs can also have a balancing action on men's energy and help prevent their bodies from becoming acidic. With an acidic body pH—which is often the result of the standard American diet—the blood can form a different kind of chi stagnation; it can become microbe- and parasite-laden, sluggish and "rusty."

Men who are vegan can risk anemia; the blood-building formulas listed in chapter seven may be helpful for them. In the following elixir, a vegan man may add dang gui to help build fresh blood. Also, men should avoid foods and liquids that produce false fire, an adrenal-derived energy that burns chi fast, leaves no fortification in its wake, and can deplete jing. These false-fire foods include, most notably, coffee and other alkaloidal drinks as well as quick-burning carbs, such as monosaccharide sugars, which are found in many sweets, pastas, and breads.

OPHIOPOGON *(mai men dong)*

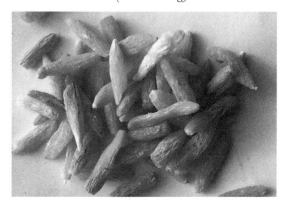

Yin replenisher,
lung yin

Herbal Elixir for Men
A Vegetarian Herbal Tea Formula for Men's Health

An anti-aging tonic to strengthen bones and upright chi, tonify kidney essence, counteract stress, enhance adaptability, and help maintain a calm yet firm disposition. Note: this tea has some herbs that mildly support sexual power.

> Ho shou wu *(Polygonum multiflorum)*: 1–2 ounces or 1 handful
> Rehmannia, prepared *(shu di huang)*: 1–2 ounces or 1 handful
> Morinda *(ba ji tian)*: 1–2 ounces or 1 handful
> Tribulus *(Bulgarus terrestrus)*: 1–2 ounces or 1 handful
> Eucommia bark *(du zhong)*: 1 ounce or 1 handful
> Astragalus *(huang chi)*: 1 ounce or 1 handful
> Chinese ginseng *(Panax quincifolium)*: 1 ounce
> Licorice root *(gan cao)*: 1 ounce or ½ handful
> Schizandra *(wu wei zi)*: 1 ounce

If you wish to build blood, add **dang gui** *(Angelica sinensis)*: 1 gram or 1 small handful.

For cooking/preparation instructions, refer to the appendix.

71

Chi Stagnation in Men

Chi stagnation in men manifests as forward distention of the belly. The classic Santa Claus look indicates chi stagnation in the form of phlegmatic buildup and the presence of parasites. Below is a picture of a man with classic chi stagnation, which affects the prostate, liver, and mood. He's been living the standard American lifestyle and eating the same way, and he is now paying the price.

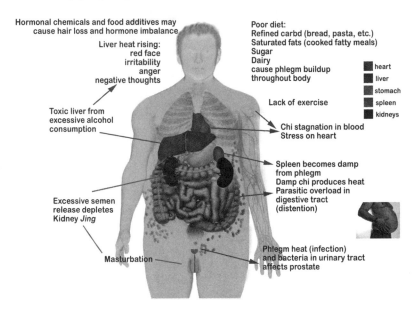

Hormonal chemicals and food additives may cause hair loss and hormone imbalance

Liver heat rising:
red face
irritability
anger
negative thoughts

Toxic liver from excessive alcohol consumption

Excessive semen release depletes Kidney *Jing*

Masturbation

Poor diet:
Refined carbd (bread, pasta, etc.)
Saturated fats (cooked fatty meals)
Sugar
Dairy
cause phlegm buildup throughout body

heart
liver
stomach
spleen
kidneys

Lack of exercise

Chi stagnation in blood
Stress on heart

Spleen becomes damp from phlegm
Damp chi produces heat
Parasitic overload in digestive tract
(distention)

Phlegm heat (infection) and bacteria in urinary tract affects prostate

This man has gathered false chi. He has major chi stagnation in the belly in the form of phlegm and parasites, which cause distention. He isn't exercising, and the chi stagnation begins to affect his urinary tract and prostate. He also releases too much semen; he is using chi to drain his jing bank. The toxicity in his body and blood is making matters worse for the liver; this manifests as "rising liver heat," which may appear as reddened skin on the face and a proverbial "hot headedness." This fella needs to do a green juice fast with blood cleansing herbal teas.

Herbs for cleansing blood, liver, and lymph include bupleurum *(chai hu)* and Scutellaria root *(huang qin)*.

BUPLEURUM (*chai hu*)

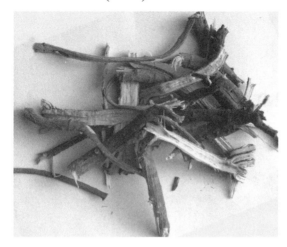

Dredge the liver,
blood, and lymph
of toxins

SCUTELLARIA (*Bicalensis*) (*huang qin*)

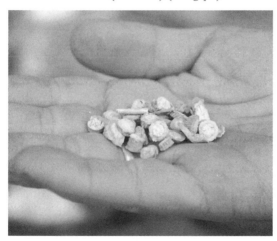

Anti-microbial,
anti-viral, nervine

Blood Cleansing Elixir for Men

In I gallon water. Drink 2–3 cups daily.

Bupleurum *(chai hu):* 2 ounces or I large handful

Scutellaria *(huang qin):* 2 ounces or I large handful

Licorice root *(gan cao):* I ounce or small handful

Ginger root (dried): 2 ounces or I handful

Astragalus *(huang chi):* 2 ounces or I large handful

White peony *(bai shao):* 2–3 ounces or I large handful

Coptis *(huang lian):* 2 grams or about 2 pieces (a very small amount is sufficient)

Taraxaci *(dandelion)*:* I once or I large handful

Gynostemma *(jiaogulan)*:* I ounce or I large handful

Schizandra *(wu wei zi)*:* I ounce or about 20–30 berries

*Add these herbs during the last three minutes of cooking.

See the appendix for cooking instructions.

Adaptogenic Herbs for Men's Health

Herbs called *adaptogens* support balanced health. They are often classified as chi, yet they have complex phytochemistry that supports chi while balancing the two branches of the nervous system; the sympathetic (defense, sexual drive, fight-or-flight) and the parasympathetic (rest, pleasure). Men are designed to thrive off acute adrenal activity, such as running from a wild tiger or chasing down an antelope. The adrenals contribute to the *yang* nature of man; therefore, adaptogenic herbs can assist the interactive forces between the two primary branches of the nervous system.

The herbs astragalus, tribulus, rhodiola, eleuthero, and morinda are very helpful adaptogenic herbs for supporting adrenal yang energy. The yang jing herb eucommia also helps fortify bone density. The formula below includes ophiopogon to add yin so that the formula is balanced and not overly yang in its effect.

Adaptogenic tea formulas can be very beneficial for men who are on the go and/or under pressure and mental or physical stress.

Adaptogenic Elixir for Men

Eleuthero root *(Siberian ginseng):* 2 ounces or 1 handful

Rhodiola *(Rhodiola crenulata):* 1–2 ounces of grated whole root or 1 gram powdered extract

Ophiopogon *(mai men dong):* 2–3 ounces or 1 handful

Astragalus *(huang chi):* 1–2 ounces or 1 handful

Chinese ginseng *(Panax quincifolium):* 1 ounce or 2 small roots, crushed

Licorice root *(gan cao):* 1 ounce or ½ handful

For cooking/preparation instructions, see the appendix.

"There are no accidents. Rather, we are moved by the silent force of evolution, which, more often than we suspect, foils our most careful plans and our expectations of staying the same. Life has evolved in adaptation to an ever-changing environment. As it attains the blossom of consciousness, it develops within each one of us the capacity to generate the changes and the lessons that will affect yet a higher adaptation and awareness."

—Michael Tierra, from *The Way of Herbs*

When we follow the way of nature, nature rewards us with a prize worth more than all the precious metals in the world—our health *and* our consciousness of it. Life begets life, and death brings on nothing more than the ash of the vessel we called home for a while. Our lives are a cosmic gift; we have been given a unique opportunity to build upon this gift and mirror God in our creativity. We can also pass on the miracle of birth—a sacred thing—and we should do everything in our power to ensure that new life thrives. This should be the simplest equation to understand, yet it remains elusive. I find it unconscionable that so many people are not given the wisdom they need to live long lives of creative and procreative empowerment. If they were, we might reach a threshold where we strive to see all life flourish, and collectively walk into the wish to thrive and to live it.

It's funny that simply learning how to eat again, and remembering how to take earth's herbal medicines, as Jesus said we should, could so easily and efficiently restore health in ourselves, our kin, and all living things we care for.

I hope to see the day when everyone realigns with the simple truth that life begets life, and in that process, Mother Nature is obeyed. She becomes our princess guardian once again. Despite our follies, she has not abandoned us, but there are definite signs that our earth is in need of our awakening. Otherwise, our support systems will lose the balanced equilibrium of chi and its collective essence, jing, which were built eons before our existence was possible.

I believe that when we reclaim a diverse seasonal and responsible dietary regimen of living foods, and when we supplement these foods with elixirs of tonic herbs for fortifying chi and jing, we will have the third "treasure," *shen;* we will become spirit children. Then, you never know, we might pierce into the grand mystery and reveal the fullness of our place in it.

Methods of Using Herbs

Preparation

Chinese tonic herbalism is reemerging as the superior herbal system. After approximately sixty years of research, Chinese medical authorities have concluded that hot water decoctions represent the best delivery system for the therapeutic properties of herbs into the body. The Chinese traditionally believed that various methods were needed to unlock the nutrients bound within the tough woody cellulose that is commonly part of Chinese herbs. These methods usually require cooking in boiling water or soaking over longer periods of time in alcohol.

The term "decoction" generally describes a long, boiled water diffusion of the herbal properties into liquid solution.

Hot Water Tea Decoction

- Fill a clay, glass, or stainless steel pot with 1 gallon water (unless otherwise specified).
- Place all herbs into the solution, with the exception of delicate herbs such as schizandra, gynostemma, mint, and magnolia flower.
- Allow the herbs to soak for twenty minutes to a half hour.
- Bring to a boil; do not over boil.
- Reduce heat to a simmer, cover, and cook for approximately one hour.
- Add delicate herbs during the last three minutes of cooking.
- Allow one to two hours to cool. Removing the pot from the stove and placing an insulated towel over the pot can help slow cooling and enhance decoction. I cover my pot and let it sit overnight. In the morning, when I remove the towel, the tea is still hot.

- Strain the tea decoction into a pitcher and place it in the refrigerator. Herbs may be placed in a separate container and refrigerated as well.
- Warm and drink two to three cups of tea daily. Sweetener, nut milk, etc., may be added for taste. This will not detract from the tea's therapeutic properties.
- Herbs may be cooked again, the same way as before. The second decoction will be less dense in taste and color, but I believe the properties of the second cooking are more yin and somewhat homeopathic.

Syrup

Herbal formulas may be decocted as concentrates. This involves cooking the herbs as described above before but for longer with no lid on the pot. Cook until the herbal tea is boiled down into a concentrate. To make a syrup, strain the tea and mix it with honey. This is an excellent way to make cough syrups or tea for children.

I once met an African herbalist who poured a spoonful of dried herb powders into the palm of my hand, then poured some honey on top and mixed it together with a Popsicle stick. He told me to lick the solution from my palm. It was a wonderful way to take the herbs!

Alcohol Decoction

The herbs in many Chinese formulas are also effective when decocted in alcohol. This method of decoction is called a *chiu*.

Place the herbs in a glass jar and add enough alcohol to submerge the herbs in the solution. Vodka, brandy, rum, or the various Chinese alcohols available in herbs shops may be used. The herbs need to soak in the alcohol for at least three months before they are ready. One ounce daily is the recommended allowance. Some of the longest living people throughout history have taken their herbs in alcohol chius, but those among us with liver damage from excessive alcohol consumption should avoid taking herbal chius.

Caution: The Chinese believe that Westerners should avoid alcohol, believing that most of us have toxic livers from over-consumption of alcoholic beverages. When taking or sharing your chiu, be cognizant of your limits. A shot or less per day is therapeutic; more may be dangerous for those with compromised livers. The Chinese believe properly combined herbal formulations in chiu may help support healthy liver function if taken in moderation.

Liquid Extract

The above process may be performed using a high-proof grain alcohol. When the herbs have been sufficiently diffused into the alcohol, you may strain out the herb residue and place the concentrate in a two- to four-ounce dropper bottle. This is a convenient way to carry the extract around in your pocket and share it with your friends.

Linaments

Certain herbal formulas may be decocted as above and massaged into to the skin as a linament. Linaments are very effective for skin inflammations and muscle aches or restless chi. Scutellaria is one of the great nervines, as are many Western herbs such as lobelia, cramp bark, hops flowers, catnip, valerian, and sassafras. These and others can be very effective when applied topically.

Selected herbs may be decocted through hot water or alcohol extraction and then skin emulsions, such as creams, vegetable glycerine, aloe vera, and coconut oil, may be added.

Jook (porridge)

One can always experiment with adding herbs to culinary dishes. A very popular and nutritious dish in China is *jook*, a rice porridge with herbs. Making jook can be a fun way to get in touch with herbal creativity. Use black, wild, and/or brown rice to make the basic porridge. Add goji, longan, codonopsis, dioscorea, jujube date, lotus seed, etc., to create a healthy meal (see Ted Kaptchuk's *The Book of Jook*).

A whole book could be written on the subject of herbal preparation/decoction, but for the sake of brevity, I'll refer you to other masters who've taken great efforts to document safe and efficacious herbal preparation techniques. Michael Tierra gives a thorough description of the various herbal processing techniques in his highly informative *The Way of Herbs* (Pocket Books, 1998) and *The Way of Chinese Herbs* (Gallery Books, 1998). James Green offers a wonderfully simple and readable exercise on herbal preparation in *The Herbal Medicine Maker's Handbook* (Crossing Press, 2000).

Sources of High-Quality Herbs

Increasing popularity is bringing excellent quality Chinese herbs closer to our homes, and we may now source high quality whole herbs and extracts online. Contact the company you are curious about and see if you can gain communication with an attentive and thoughtful representative. I find that TCM herbalists are usually interested in talking about the details of herbology and may happily offer many fruitful conversations to help guide you to the best herbs for your needs. I also have an online course on tonic herbalism and Taoist health philosophy that offers helpful insights on herb sourcing: www.gateoflife.org.

Dragon Herbs
Ron Teeguarden
315 Wilshire Blvd.
Santa Monica, CA 90401
(888) 55-TONIC

Beverly Hills
460 S. Robertson Blvd.
Los Angeles, CA 90048
(310) 860-8945

Jing Herbs
George Lamoureaux
533 Los Angeles St. #502
Los Angeles, CA 90013
(213) 873-4488

Tonix Botanical Solutions
Desiree Romero
desiree@mytonix.com
(213) 280-8310

The Forgotten Foods . . . Remembered
Baratunde & Kayah Ma'at-Alexander
Atlanta, GA
longlife@theforgottenfoods.com
(770) 573-0488

Shaman Shack Herbs
www.shamanshackherbs.com
(323) 423-3207
Contact: Brynn Booth, shamanshackbrynn@gmail.com

Gate of Life
Rehmannia Dean Thomas's online course on tonic herbalism
    and Taoist health philosophy
www.GateofLife.org

Mountain Rose Herbs grows some excellent wildcrafted
    and organic bulk herbs, including many Chinese herbs.
P.O. Box 50220
Eugene, OR 97405
(800) 879-3337

Mayway Co. in Oakland, California, is an excellent supplier
    of whole bulk Chinese herbs, extracts and formulas.
(800) 2 MAYWAY

1. This comparison of chi and ATP is my own observation. I have not read a technical comparison anywhere, and I doubt one exists. The exact mechanisms may be slightly different, but I believe they are essentially the same.

2. N. W. Walker. *Raw Vegetable Juices* (Boynton Beach, FL: Pyramid, 1936).

3. Oliver Morton. *Eating the Sun: How Plants Power the Planet* (New York: Harper Collins, 2007), 158.

4. Dan Koontz, Jack Hinze, et al., "Leaky Gut Syndrome (LGS) Origins, Effects and Therapies, The 'Medical Link' Between Dysbiosis and Many Major Ailments, 'Is This the Most Misdiagnosed/Underdiagnosed Condition in Medicine Today?'" *The Herbal Pharm* 19 (1999): 8.

5. Leo Galland, "Dysbiotic Relationships in the Bowel." American College of Advancement in Medicine Conference, Spring 1992.

6. C. P. Tamboli, C. Neut, et al., "Dysbiosis in inflammatory bowel disease." *Gut* (January 2004); 53 (1): 1–4.

7. Antonio Tursi, Giovanni Bradimarte, et al., "Assessment of small intestinal bacterial overgrowth in uncomplicated acute diverticulitis of the colon." *World Journal of Gastroenterology* (June 2005); 11 (18): 2773–6.

8. Natasha Campbell-McBride. *Gut and Psychology Syndrome: Natural Treatment for Autism, Dyspraxia, A.D.D., Dyslexia, A.D.H.D., Depression, Schizophrenia.* (Medinform Publishing 2010).

9. William G. Crook. "Sugar, yeast and ADHD: fact or fiction?" in Joseph A. Bellanti, William G. Crook et al., eds, Attention Deficit Hyperactivity Disorder: Causes and Possible Solutions (Proceedings of a Conference). (Jackson, TN: International Health Foundation: 1999.)

10. Leo Galland, "Nutritional Supplementation for ADHD" in Joseph A.

Bellanti, William G. Crook et al., eds, Attention Deficit Hyperactivity Disorder: Causes and Possible Solutions (Proceedings of a Conference). (Jackson, TN: International Health Foundation: 1999.)

11. Horace Kephart and Ralph Roberts, *Our Southern Highlanders* (New York: Outing Publishing, 1913), 39.

12. Michael Tierra, *The Way of Chinese Herbs* (New York: Pocket Books, 1980).

13. Dan Bensky and Andrew Gamble, *Chinese Herbal Medicine Materia Medica* (Seattle, Washington: Eastland Press, 1986), 322.

14. Ibid.

15. I. I. Brekhman and I. V. Dardymov, "New Substances of Plant Origin which Increase Nonspecific Resistance." *Annual Review of Pharmacology* 9 (1969): 419–430, doi:10.1146/annurev.pa.09 .040169.002223.

16. Michael Blumert and Jialiu Liu, *Jiaogulan: China's "Immortality" Herb* (Badger, California: Torchlight Publishing, 1999).

17. Subhuti Dharmananda, "Safety Issues Affecting Chinese Herbs: The Case of Ginseng," www.itm-online.org/arts/ginseng.htm.

ABOUT THE AUTHOR

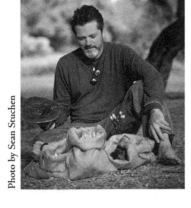

Photo by Sean Stuchen

REHMANNIA DEAN THOMAS is a Taoist tonic herbalist in the Gate of Life Lineage, a 5,000-year-old health system from China that utilizes tonic herbs to help maintain overall health of the body, mind, and spirit. He completed an eight-year traditional master-pupil apprenticeship under Master Herbalist Ron Teeguarden and studied traditional Chinese medicine diagnosis at Alhambra University. He holds a degree as Master Herbalist from Natural Healing College. He has created an online course on Taoist herbology, www.gateoflife.org. Originally from Louisville, Kentucky, he now resides in Upland, California.